Endocrinology

Editors

MICHAEL MALONE
VASUDHA JAIN

PRIMARY CARE: CLINICS IN OFFICE PRACTICE

www.primarycare.theclinics.com

Consulting Editor
JOEL J. HEIDELBAUGH

September 2024 • Volume 51 • Number 3

ELSEVIER

1600 John F. Kennedy Boulevard • Suite 1800 • Philadelphia, Pennsylvania, 19103-2899

http://www.theclinics.com

PRIMARY CARE: CLINICS IN OFFICE PRACTICE Volume 51, Number 3
September 2024 ISSN 0095-4543, ISBN-13: 978-0-443-29382-5

Editor: Taylor Hayes
Developmental Editor: Nitesh Barthwal

Primary Care: Clinics in Office Practice (ISSN: 0095-4543) is published quarterly by Elsevier Inc., 360 Park Avenue South, New York, NY 10010-1710. Months of issue are March, June, September, and December. Periodicals postage paid at New York, NY and additional mailing offices. Subscription prices are $277.00 per year (US individuals), $100.00 (US students), $331.00 (Canadian individuals), $100.00 (Canadian students), $390.00 (international individuals), and $175.00 (international students). For institutional access pricing please contact Customer Service via the contact information below. Foreign air speed delivery is included in all *Clinics* subscription prices. All prices are subject to change without notice. Orders, claims, and journal inquiries: Please visit our Support Hub page https://service.elsevier.com for assistance.

Reprints. For copies of 100 or more, of articles in this publication, please contact the Commercial Reprints Department, Elsevier Inc., 360 Park Avenue South, New York, NY 10010-1710. Tel. 212-633-3874; Fax: 212-633-3820; E-mail: reprints@elsevier.com.

Primary Care: Clinics in Office Practice is covered in *MEDLINE/PubMed (Index Medicus)* and *EMBASE/ Excerpta Medica, Current Contents/Clinical Medicine,* and *ISI/BIOMED.*

Contributors

CONSULTING EDITOR

JOEL J. HEIDELBAUGH, MD, FAAFP, FACG
Clinical Professor, Departments of Family Medicine and Urology, Director of Medical Student Education and Clerkship Director, Department of Family Medicine, University of Michigan Medical School, Ann Arbor, Michigan; Ypsilanti Health Center, Ypsilanti, Michigan

EDITORS

MICHAEL MALONE, MD
Program Director, Tidelands Health MUSC Family Medicine Residency, Designated Institutional Official for GME, Tidelands Health, Department of Family Medicine, Tidelands Health Family Medicine Residency Program, Tidelands Health with MUSC Health, Murrells Inlet, Myrtle Beach, South Carolina

VASUDHA JAIN, MD
Assistant Program Director and Core Faculty, Tidelands Health MUSC Family Medicine Residency, Designated Institutional Official, Medical Director, Department of Family Medicine, Tidelands Health with MUSC Health, Myrtle Beach, South Carolina

AUTHORS

THERESE ANDERSON, MD
Clinical Instructor, Consultant, Department of Family Medicine, Mayo Clinic, Jacksonville, Florida

SHEHAR BANO AWAIS, MD
Family Medicine Physician, WellSpan Good Samaritan Hospital Family Medicine Residency Program, Lebanon, Pennsylvania

REBECCA BOWIE, MD
Resident Physician, Family Medicine Doctor, Department of Family Medicine, Mayo Clinic, Jacksonville, Florida

GAURI DHIR, MD, FACC
Physician, Department of Endocrinology, Tidelands Health System, Murrells Inlet, South Carolina

TYLER FULLER, MD
Resident Physician, Department of Family and Community Medicine, Penn State University College of Medicine, Milton S. Hershey Medical Center, Hershey, Pennsylvania

LESLIE A. GREENBERG, MD, FAAFP
Associate Professor, Department of Family and Community Medicine, University of Nevada Reno School of Medicine, Reno, Nevada

FRANCIS GUERRA-BAUMAN, MD
Family Medicine Doctor, Department of Family Medicine, WellSpan Good Samaritan
Hospital Family Medicine Residency Program, Lebanon, Pennsylvania

CHRISTINA T. HANOS, MD
Chief Resident, Department of Family Medicine, Mayo Clinic, Jacksonville, Florida

VASUDHA JAIN, MD
Assistant Program Director and Core Faculty, Tidelands Health MUSC Family
Medicine Residency, Designated Institutional Official, Medical Director, Department
of Family Medicine, Tidelands Health with MUSC Health, Myrtle Beach, South
Carolina

TYLER M. JANITZ, DO
Resident, Department of Family Medicine, Mayo Clinic, Jacksonville, Florida

KATHERINE JOHNSON, MD
Physician, Diplomate of ABOM, Diplomate of ABCL, Department of Family Medicine, Self
Regional Healthcare, Greenwood, South Carolina

SUKHJEET KAMBOJ, MD, FAAFP
Associate Professor and Interim Program Director, Department of Family Medicine,
WellSpan Good Samaritan Hospital Family Medicine Residency Program, Lebanon,
Pennsylvania

RAMLA N. KASOZI, MB, CHB, MPH
Family Medicine Physician, Department of Family Medicine, Mayo Clinic, Jacksonville,
Florida

HENRY LAU, DO, FAAFP
Associate Program Director, Department of Family Medicine, Tidelands Health, Myrtle
Beach, South Carolina

MEGAN ILENE LAUGHREY, MD
Resident Physician, Department of Family Medicine, Tidelands Health Medical University
of South Carolina Residency Program, Myrtle Beach, South Carolina

KESWICK LO, MD
Family Medicine Resident Physician, Department of Family Medicine, Tidelands Health,
Myrtle Beach, South Carolina

HUSSAIN MAHMUD, MD
Assistant Professor, Endocrinology Division, Department of Medicine, UPMC Center for
Endocrinology & Metabolism, Associate Program Director, Endocrinology Fellowship,
University of Pittsburgh Medical College, UPMC Center for Endocrinology and
Metabolism, Pittsburgh, Pennsylvania

MICHAEL MALONE, MD
Program Director, Tidelands Health MUSC Family Medicine Residency, Designated
Institutional Official for GME, Tidelands Health, Department of Family Medicine, Tidelands
Health Family Medicine Residency Program, Tidelands Health with MUSC Health,
Murrells Inlet, Myrtle Beach, South Carolina

MATTHEW McCOSKEY, MD
Core Faculty Physician, Department of Family Medicine, Tidelands Health, Myrtle Beach,
South Carolina

SHELBY MCGEE, DO
Family Medicine Resident Physician, Department of Family Medicine, Tidelands Health, Myrtle Beach, South Carolina

ANDREW MERRITT, MD
PGY-2 Resident, Department of Family Medicine, Tidelands Health Family Medicine Residency Program, Myrtle Beach, South Carolina

MUNIMA NASIR, MD
Associate Professor, Department of Family and Community Medicine, Penn State University College of Medicine, Milton S. Hershey Medical Center, Hershey, Pennsylvania

ZAKARY NEWBERRY, MD
Resident Physician, Department of Family and Community Medicine, Penn State University College of Medicine, Milton S. Hershey Medical Center, Hershey, Pennsylvania

MARK OWOLABI, MD
Family Medicine Physician, Department of Family Medicine, MedStar Georgetown University Hospital, Medstar Health, Georgetown-Washington Hospital Center, Washington, DC

JUAN A. PEREZ, DO
Assistant Professor, Department of Family and Community Medicine Residency Program, Penn State Health St. Joseph Medical Center, Reading, Pennsylvania

GEORGE G.A. PUJALTE, MD
Associate Professor, Departments of Family Medicine and Orthopedic Surgery, Mayo Clinic, Jacksonville, Florida

SARAH INÉS RAMÍREZ, MD, FAAFP
Associate Professor, Department of Family and Community Medicine, Penn State University College of Medicine, Hershey, Pennsylvania

LARAE L. SEEMANN, MD
Chief Resident, Department of Family Medicine, Mayo Clinic, Jacksonville, Florida

MONICA SELANDER-HAN, DO
Obstetrics and Gynecology Specialist, Department of Family Medicine, Tidelands Health, Myrtle Beach, South Carolina

ALEC SIKARIN, MD
Resident, Department of Family Medicine, Tidelands Health, Myrtle Beach, South Carolina

ELIZABETH ASHLEY SUNIEGA, MD
Family Medicine Doctor, Department of Family Medicine, Tidelands Health Medical University of South Carolina Residency Program, Myrtle Beach, South Carolina

JUSTIN TONDT, MD
Assistant Professor, Department of Family and Community Medicine, Penn State University College of Medicine, Milton S. Hershey Medical Center, Hershey, Pennsylvania

ANNA VAN NIEKERK, DO
Clinical Instructor, Family Medicine Doctor, Department of Family Medicine, Mayo Clinic, Jacksonville, Florida

NICHOLAS VERNON, DO
Family Medicine Resident - PGY3, Department of Family Medicine, Tidelands Health,
Myrtle Beach, South Carolina

ABDUL WAHEED, MD, MS PHS, CPE, FAAFP
Professor and Chair, Department of Family Medicine, Dignity Health Medical Group,
Creighton University School of Medicine, Phoenix, Arizona

Contents

different endocrine tumors affecting primarily the parathyroid glands, gastroenteropancreatic tract, and the anterior pituitary gland. Multiple endocrine neoplasia type 2A (MEN2A) and Multiple endocrine neoplasia type 2B (MEN2B) are autosomal dominant genetic syndromes because of a germline variant in the 'rearranged during transfection' (RET) proto-oncogene. There are common RET mutations causing receptor hyperactivation and induction of downstream signals that cause oncogenesis. Common conditions with MEN2A are medullary thyroid cancer (MTC), pheochromocytoma, and primary hyperparathyroidism. Common conditions with MEN2B include MTC, pheochromocytomas, and benign ganglioneuromas.

Endocrine Emergencies   495

Abdul Waheed, Shehar Bano Awais, Sukhjeet Kamboj, and Hussain Mahmud

Endocrine emergencies encompass a group of conditions that occur when hormonal deficiency or excess results in acute presentation. If these endocrine disorders are not rapidly identified or if specific treatment is delayed, significant complications or even death may occur. This article outlines the basics of endocrine emergencies involving the thyroid, parathyroid, pituitary, pancreas, and adrenal glands. It discusses various causative factors, diagnostic approaches, and treatment modalities, emphasizing the significance of preventive measures. This article is aimed at guiding health care professionals, and this overview seeks to enhance understanding and improve patient outcomes in managing endocrine emergencies.

Obesity   511

Tyler Fuller, Zakary Newberry, Munima Nasir, and Justin Tondt

Obesity is a complex, multifactorial disease that is highly prevalent in the United States. Obesity is typically classified by body mass index and the US Preventive Services Task Force recommends screening all patients 6 years or older for obesity. Evaluation includes a thorough history and physical examination as well as laboratory tests including hemoglobin A1c, comprehensive metabolic panel, lipid panel, and thyroid-stimulating hormone. Treatment involves a multidisciplinary approach including nutrition, physical activity, and behavioral therapy as well as pharmacotherapy and bariatric surgery when appropriate.

Sports Endocrinology   523

Henry Lau, Tyler M. Janitz, Alec Sikarin, Ramla N. Kasozi, and George G.A. Pujalte

Sports endocrinology holds a unique importance in understanding and optimizing an active and healthy lifestyle. Active patients with diabetes will need to consider modifying medications, especially insulin. The use of the dual energy x-ray absorptiometry and Fracture Risk Assessment Tool scores is important as both initiate and monitor bone health treatment. Menstrual disorders and energy imbalances are some special concerns when treating female athletes, calling for a multidisciplinary treatment team. Performance agents are popular and have made their way into recreational sports.

Disequilibrium of hormonal intercommunication between the maternal brain and the developing fetal–placental unit increases morbidity and mortality risk for the mother–baby dyad. As a novel yet temporary endocrine organ, the placenta serves as a physical and immunologic barrier that facilitates exchange of nutrients and elimination of fetal waste. Steroid and peptide-based hormones secreted by the placenta and other neuroendocrine organs induce adaptations in maternal physiology accommodating fetal growth and development and enabling lactation postpartum. Human placental growth hormone, a peptide hormone continuously secreted at increasing concentrations throughout pregnancy, is a primary determinant of maternal insulin resistance and gestational diabetes.

Neuroendocrine neoplasms (NENs), also known as neuroendocrine tumors (NETs), are rare tumors derived from cells with characteristics of both nerve and endocrine cells. The clinical presentation, diagnosis, and treatment of NENs vary significantly depending on the type, location, whether the neoplasm is hormonally functional, how aggressive it is, and whether it has metastasized to other parts of the body. This article provides an overview of specific types of NETs, clinical presentations and related syndromes, diagnosis, and approach to management of common NENs.

PRIMARY CARE:
CLINICS IN OFFICE PRACTICE

SERIES OF RELATED INTEREST

Medical Clinics (http://www.medical.theclinics.com)
Physician Assistant Clinics (https://www.physicianassistant.theclinics.com)

THE CLINICS ARE AVAILABLE ONLINE!
Access your subscription at:
www.theclinics.com

PRIMARY CARE
CLINICS IN OFFICE PRACTICE

FORTHCOMING ISSUES

December 2024
Adolescent Medicine
Amanda B. Kost and Kerry Popielec, Editors

March 2025
Ear, Nose, and Throat Issues in Primary Care
Donna M. Kemmati, Editor

June 2025
Women's Health
Sarina Schrager and Heather Paladine, Editors

RECENT ISSUES

June 2024
Neurology
Kara Wyatt and Melissa Elafros, Editors

March 2024
Cardiovascular Diseases
Anthony Viera, Editor

December 2023
Social Determinants of Health
Vincent Morelli and Joel J. Heidelbaugh, Editors

SERIES OF RELATED INTEREST

Medical Clinics (http://www.medical.theclinics.com)
Physician Assistant Clinics (https://www.physicianassistant.theclinics.com)

THE CLINICS ARE AVAILABLE ONLINE!
Access your subscription at:
www.theclinics.com

Foreword

New Drugs, New Strategies, New Demand

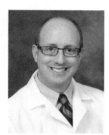

Joel J. Heidelbaugh, MD, FAAFP, FACG
Consulting Editor

The field of endocrinology presents diagnostic challenges that span multiple organs and organ systems, hormones and electrolytes, and symptoms both concrete and vague. Recent years have seen the advent of new drug classes and treatment strategies, including the glucagon-like peptide-1 (GLP-1) agonists used to treat diabetes mellitus and obesity. These medications are some of the most extensively prescribed (and extensively coveted) drugs on the market today. Demand far exceeds supply. Patients who are suitable candidates often have to work through prior authorizations; analogues are being rapidly compounded, and some patients who were started on these medications can no longer get them due to supply shortages or changes in insurance coverage. While this is a landmark breakthrough in treatment for diabetes and obesity, with more indications for the GLP-1 agonists arising on a near monthly basis, the opportunity for widespread prescription comes with great challenges. Moreover, treatment controversies persist within endocrinology, especially in the realm of male hormone replacement.

An article published in 2020 that studied trends in the endocrinologist workforce revealed some shocking details.[1] The approximate 50% expansion in endocrinology training positions from 223 in 2009 to 326 in 2019 was accompanied by a stagnant number of applications with an applicant/position ratio approaching 1.0. In addition to attrition primarily due to retirement, the number of filled endocrinology fellowship positions has not adequately populated the need for practicing endocrinologists to care for our expanding and aging population. The perceived likelihood of poor job satisfaction as a measure of the balance of workload, lifestyle, compensation, professional development, and relationship with patients seems to outweigh the intellectual stimulation and value of longitudinal relationship with patients. As an essentially "nonprocedural"-based field, endocrinology has the lowest compensation among subspecialties, and

Prim Care Clin Office Pract 51 (2024) xiii–xiv
https://doi.org/10.1016/j.pop.2024.06.002
0095-4543/24/© 2024 Published by Elsevier Inc.

increasing time spent on paperwork and the exponential pressure to see more patients are major disincentives to recruit future endocrinologists. All of these factors seemingly drive primary care clinicians to be more adept at the diagnosis and management of common endocrinology disorders.

This issue of *Primary Care: Clinics in Office Practice* dedicated to endocrinology is extensively comprehensive and highlights current evidence-based guidelines on many common disorders we encounter in our practices. It covers "the common topics," and the "nuts-and-bolts" information is presented in a very useful fashion but also presents articles on endocrine emergencies, sports endocrinology, and endocrinology during pregnancy. I would like to thank Drs Michael Malone and Vasudha Jain for compiling this outstanding issue, as well as the many authors who wrote outstanding and practical articles. I hope that you will find this issue of *Primary Care: Clinics in Office Practice* to be as informative as I have found it to be.

Joel J. Heidelbaugh, MD, FAAFP, FACG
Departments of Family Medicine and Urology
University of Michigan Medical School
Ann Arbor, MI 48103, USA

Ypsilanti Health Center
200 Arnet, Suite 200
Ypsilanti, MI 48198, USA

E-mail address:
jheidel@umich.edu

REFERENCE

1. Romeo GR, Hirsch IB, Lash RW, et al. Trends in the endocrinology fellowship recruitment: reasons for concern and possible interventions. J Clin Endocrinol Metab 2020;105(6):1701–6.

Preface

Endocrinology in Primary Care

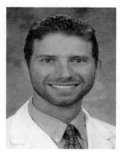 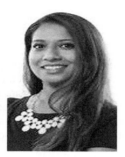

Michael Malone, MD   Vasudha Jain, MD
Editors

Primary Care Providers are the initial or continuity provider for many patients with endocrine conditions. Therefore, an up-to-date high-quality medical reference tailored specifically for primary care is necessary. We are pleased to offer this issue of *Primary Care: Clinics in Office Practice* devoted to endocrine disorders. The fourteen topics covered in this issue were thoughtfully selected to address conditions that are highly relevant for primary care. Each topic was then organized and written in a way that can be easily utilized by clinicians in a busy clinical setting.

Many endocrine disorders have a significant delay between the time of initial presentation to a physician and diagnosis. This delay in diagnosis is likely because endocrine conditions can present with vague symptoms primary care providers can attribute to nonendocrine conditions. The symptoms of endocrine disorders are seen commonly, often daily, in primary care. These symptoms include mood and cognitive changes, elevated blood pressure, elevated blood sugar, headache, menstrual irregularities, electrolyte disturbances, disruption of thermoregulation, changes in bone mineral density, and fatigue. We hope this issue allows primary providers to reduce the current delay in the diagnosis of endocrine disorders by increasing their comfort and knowledge of endocrine conditions.

Each article is structured to provide a practical reference with evidence-based guidance on assessment and treatment options for common endocrine topics. Some of the topics in this issue include pituitary disorders, adrenal disorders, endocrine tumors, endocrine emergencies, sports endocrinology, and reproductive disorders. We hope you enjoy reading this issue and think you will find it evidence-based and clinically relevant for primary care.

Prim Care Clin Office Pract 51 (2024) xv–xvi
https://doi.org/10.1016/j.pop.2024.06.001
0095-4543/24/© 2024 Published by Elsevier Inc.   **primarycare.theclinics.com**

DISCLOSURES

The authors have no conflicts of interest to disclose.

Michael Malone, MD
Tidelands Health MUSC Family Medicine Residency
Department of Family Medicine
Tidelands Health with MUSC Health
4320 Holmestown Road
Myrtle Beach, SC 29588, USA

Vasudha Jain, MD
Tidelands Health MUSC Family Medicine Residency
Department of Family Medicine
Tidelands Health with MUSC Health
4320 Holmestown Road
Myrtle Beach, SC 29588, USA

E-mail addresses:
mimalone@tidelandshealth.org (M. Malone)
vjain@tidelandshealth.org (V. Jain)

Glucose Disorders

Juan A. Perez, DO

KEYWORDS

- Insulin resistance • Diabetes mellitus type 2 • Gestational diabetes mellitus • MODY
- Diabetes mellitus type 1 • LADA • Cushing's • Atypical antipsychotics

KEY POINTS

- Primary conditions causing hyperglycemia are often overlapping syndromes characterized by insulin resistance, defective insulin production or release, and autoimmune destruction of the pancreatic islet cells.
- Secondary causes of hyperglycemia include various endocrine disorders and medication or drug-induced infections.
- Hypoglycemia can be due to states of glucose underproduction: Hormone/enzyme deficiencies and acquired liver diseases.
- Hypoglycemia may also result from conditions causing glucose overconsumption such as hyperinsulinism or metabolic deficiencies.
- Inherited disorders of glucose and glycogen metabolism constitute a small percentage of glucose disorders.

HYPERGLYCEMIA
Introduction

Hyperglycemia is defined as an elevation of blood glucose. It is often related to defective insulin production or release, insulin resistance, or autoimmune destruction of the pancreatic islet cells.

Hyperglycemia due to Insulin Resistance

Insulin resistance is an impaired biologic response to insulin stimulation of target tissues. Insulin resistance can cause prediabetes and as it worsens leads to Type II diabetes mellitus (T2DM). The risk factors for insulin resistance are the same as for T2DM and include family history, former gestational diabetes mellitus (DM), older age, polycystic ovarian syndrome (PCOS), visceral obesity, sedentary lifestyle, and non-Caucasian ethnicity[1]

A constellation of conditions known as metabolic syndrome can occur with insulin resistance. The World Health Organization defines metabolic syndrome as having 3 or more of the following traits listed in **Table 1**.[2]

Department of Family and Community Medicine Residency Program, Penn State Health-St. Joseph Hospital, 145 N. 6th Street, 2nd floor, Reading, PA 19601, USA
E-mail address: jperez8@pennstatehealth.psu.edu

Prim Care Clin Office Pract 51 (2024) 375–390
https://doi.org/10.1016/j.pop.2024.03.003
0095-4543/24/© 2024 Elsevier Inc. All rights reserved.
primarycare.theclinics.com

Table 1 Metabolic Syndrome Criteria	
Increased waist circumference	> 40″ in men, > 35″ in women
Increased triglycerides	≥ 150 mg/dL
Decreased high-density lipoprotein	< 40 mg/dL in men, < 50 mg/dL in women
Elevated fasting blood glucose	>100 mg/dL
Elevated blood pressure	≥ 130/85 mm Hg

Insulin resistance is also associated with elevated inflammatory markers, endothelial dysfunction, and a prothrombotic state.[3]

Hyperglycemia due to Reduced Insulin Production

Reduced insulin production leading to insulin deficiency is usually due to autoimmune destruction of the pancreatic islet cells, as is the case in Type I DM (T1DM).

Symptoms of Hyperglycemia

Signs and symptoms of hyperglycemia include polyuria, polydipsia, weight loss, fatigue, blurry vision, neuropathy, and frequent infections (particularly genitourinary candidal).

Evaluation of Hyperglycemia

Initial screening laboratory tests for hyperglycemia include fasting glucose, random glucose, and/or A1C. Once hyperglycemia is confirmed, further testing varies based on the likely etiologies.

There are multiple conditions that can alter the accuracy of A1C results. Hemolytic anemias, acute blood loss, pregnancy, antiretroviral therapies, and chronic liver disease can falsely lower A1C results.[4,5] Splenectomy, aplastic anemias, iron-deficiency anemias, renal failure, hyperbilirubinemia, and hypertriglyceridemia can falsely elevate A1C values.[4,5] Hemoglobinopathies and hemoglobin variants can result in variable changes in A1C measurements, A1C results are commonly falsely low.[4,5]

Secondary Causes of Hyperglycemia

Endocrine disorders
Acromegaly is caused by elevated growth hormone (GH) in an adult. Chronic GH excess impairs insulin sensitivity, increases gluconeogenesis, reduces the glucose uptake in adipose tissue and muscle, and alters pancreatic β-cell function.[6]

Glucagonoma are neuroendocrine tumors that occur in the pancreas and lead to excess glucagon production. The elevated glucagon leads to increased gluconeogenesis which induces a hyperglycemic state.

Thyrotoxicosis is due to excess circulating thyroid hormones and is associated with poor glycemic control, including hyperglycemia and insulinopenia. Up to half of those with Graves' disease will develop some degree of glucose intolerance and approximately 2% to 3% individuals with hyperthyroidism develop overt diabetes.[7]

Cushing's syndrome is due to increased production of cortisol (the stress hormone). Cortisol exacerbates gluconeogenesis and hepatic glucose output through both direct and indirect effects.[5,8] Chronic glucocorticoid exposure also induces selective insulin resistance that impedes the inhibitory effect of insulin on hepatic glucose output.[8]

Pheochromocytoma is a neuroendocrine tumor producing an excess of catecholamines (epinephrine, norepinephrine, dopamine) and can induce insulin resistance.[9]

Medication/drug induced

Medications associated with hyperglycemia include glucocorticoids, atypical antipsychotics, calcineurin inhibitors, protease inhibitors, thiazides, niacin, and statins.[10-12]

Pancreatic disease

Chronic pancreatitis, cystic fibrosis, or pancreatic cancer may damage the pancreatic beta-cells, thus reducing insulin production and resulting in diabetes mellitus.

Insulin Receptor Antibodies is a rare cause of insulin resistance. Patients with this condition can present with hyperglycemia, insulin resistance, and acanthosis nigricans.[13]

Genetic syndromes

Hemochromatosis causes iron deposition in the pancreas which can damage beta-cells and reduce insulin production.

Cystic fibrosis can lead to pancreatic disease affecting both exocrine and endocrine functions of the pancreas.

Physiologic stress

Injury, sepsis, and surgery can all induce transient hyperglycemia.

Complications of Hyperglycemia

Acute and subacute complications of hyperglycemia include diabetic ketoacidosis (DKA) and hyperglycemic hyperosmolar state (HHS). Left untreated, fatal cerebral edema can occur in both conditions, but is more common in DKA. Chronic possible complications from hyperglycemia include both microvascular ones: retinopathy, nephropathy, neuropathy and macrovascular complications: coronary artery disease, cerebrovascular disease, and peripheral vascular disease.[14]

PREDIABETES
Definition

The American Diabetic Association (ADA) defines prediabetes as having elevated fasting glucose in the 100 to 125 mg/dL range or an A1C value of 5.7% to 6.4%.[15]

Prevalence

It is estimated that 96 million people in the United States have prediabetes (38% of the adult US population).[16]

Risk Factors

Age and body mass index (BMI) are 2 of the strongest risk factors for prediabetes; evidence has demonstrated a strong age-related increase in pre-diabetes.[17]

The ADA risk screening tool uses 6 criteria: age, gender, family history, history of high blood pressure, physical activity level, and BMI.[18]

Clinical Features

Prediabetes is typically asymptomatic. Patients with prediabetes usually have an increased BMI and may have acanthosis nigricans. Clinical features of prediabetes related to PCOS include insulin resistance, secondary amenorrhea, obesity, and hyperandrogenism.

Screening

The US Preventive Services Task Force (USPSTF) (August 24, 2021-GRADE B) recommends screening for prediabetes and type 2 diabetes in adults aged 35 to 70 years who are overweight (BMI >25) or obese (BMI >30).

Therapeutic Options

Lifestyle approaches with increased exercise, reducing carbohydrates, and decreasing weight is the cornerstone of treatments for insulin resistance. Insulin-sensitizing medications such as the biguanides (metformin) and GLP-1 receptor agonists can also be utilized.

DIABETES MELLITUS TYPE 2
Definition

Criteria for diagnosis[19]

HbA1C >6.4%, fasting plasma glucose ≥126 mg/dL, and random plasma glucose ≥200 mg/dL.

Prevalence

A total of 28.7 million people of all ages—or 8.7% of the US population have diagnosed diabetes.

A total of 8.5 million people (23% of diabetics) have undiagnosed diabetes.
A total of 11.3% of the US population is diabetic.[16]

Pathogenesis

Insulin resistance and a progressive loss of beta-cell function.

Evaluation and Diagnosis

The evaluation of Type II DM includes confirming an elevated glucose state and insulin resistance. To differentiate between Type I and Type II DM, it is helpful to obtain a C-peptide and pancreatic antibodies.[20,21] The antibodies are commonly run as a panel of Islet-cell antibodies, antibodies to insulin, glutamic acid decarboxylase antibodies, and protein tyrosine phosphatase antibodies. In most case, islet-cell antibody testing is sufficient as it is the most sensitive and specific.[20,21]

C-peptide is a marker for endogenous insulin production. Therefore, normal or elevated c-peptide levels with negative antibodies are consistent with insulin resistance and Type II DM.[17] The absence or extremely low levels of c-peptide with positive pancreatic antibodies confirms the diagnosis of Type I DM.[22]

Clinical Features

Overlapping with metabolic syndrome and PCOS, patients commonly present with an elevated BMI (>25), acanthosis nigricans, hypertension, dyslipidemia, and fatty liver disease. Most will be asymptomatic initially. Significant hyperglycemia causes glycosuria and thus an osmotic diuresis leading to urinary frequency, polyuria, and polydipsia that may progress to orthostatic hypotension and dehydration. Severe dehydration causes weakness, fatigue, and mental status changes. Hyperglycemia can also cause weight loss, nausea and vomiting, blurred vision, and it may also predispose to bacterial or fungal infections.[23]

Acute and Chronic Complications

Acute complications include hyperosmolar hyperglycemic coma.

Chronic complications are both microvascular and macrovascular and include diabetic retinopathy, nephropathy/renal disease, diabetic peripheral neuropathy, peripheral vascular disease, and cardiovascular disease. Tight glucose control in DM2 prevents long-term microvascular complications, although the benefits on macrovascular outcomes are not as robust.

Treatment Goals

Target A1C goals between 6.0% and 9.0% and need to be individualized to each patient. Treatment goals vary based on age, life expectancy, presence of comorbidities, patient preference and resources, disease duration, presence of diabetic complications, and the risk of hypoglycemia or other adverse side effects.[19] Very tight glucose control in the elderly may lead increased morbidity and mortality due to hypoglycemia, falls, increased risk of dementia, and cardiac arrhythmias.[24]

Continuous Glucose Monitors

Continuous glucose monitors (CGMs) allow for real-time glucose monitoring with alerts transmitted to patients during times of rising or falling glucose levels. Certain CGMs can also be integrated with an insulin pump, which allows the monitor to automatically adjust or pause insulin delivery in response to any significant change in glucose.[25]

Therapeutic Options

Non-medication therapies

Lifestyle changes including increased exercise and weight loss remain the cornerstone of early DM2 treatment and should be maintained even after the introduction of medication therapy.[26] Weight loss is highly beneficial for diabetes control. For those with a significantly elevated BMI, bariatric surgery may induce remission of DM.[27]

MEDICATIONS

Metformin remains the standard first-line medicine due to safety, cost, and insulin-sensitizing properties. Newer agents such as the SGLT-2 inhibitors and GLP-1 agonists also have the added cardioprotective and weight loss (GLP-1) benefits, and may be considered first line treatments in the presence of coexisting cardiovascular disease and/or elevated BMI. For non-insulin medication options, please refer to **Table 2**.[28,29]

Insulin is indicated when oral medications are contraindicated or when the patient is uncontrolled on multiple non-insulin medications. The ADA suggests the use of basal insulin to augment therapy when the A1C is 9% or more.[30] For diabetics with blood glucose level greater than 300 mg/dL or the A1C > 10%, the ADA suggests insulin replacement therapy with both basal and prandial insulin as the primary treatment modality.[30] The American Association of Clinical Endocrinologists and the American College of Endocrinology guidelines recommend augmenting treatment with basal insulin when the A1C is more than 8%.[31] For the different types of insulins and their properties, refer to **Table 3**.

Cost is based on information obtained at http://www.goodrx.com (accessed October 15, 2023) and calculated on a per unit basis based on retail price without discounts (**Table 4**).

$ = less than $0.1/unit.
$$ = $0.1 to $0.19/unit.
$$$ = $0.2 to $0.29/unit.
$$$$ = over $0.3/unit.

DIABETES MELLITUS TYPE 1
Definition

In Type I DM, autoimmune beta-cell destruction leads to decreased insulin production in pancreas and ultimately to hyperglycemia due to insulin deficiency. A laboratory test

Table 2
Non-insulin medication classes for diabetes mellitus in chronologic order of their Food and Drug Administration approval date (first medicine in class), primary mode of action, adverse effects, and cost

Medication Class and Year Approved[b]	Primary Mode of Action	Adverse Effects	Cost[a]
Sulfonylureas: 1984 (glipizide, glyburide, glimepiride)	Secretagogues: stimulate B-cell insulin release	Hypoglycemia, weight gain	$
Biguanides: 1995 (metformin)	Decrease hepatic glucose output, increase peripheral glucose uptake (sensitizer)	Diarrhea, bloating. Lactic acidosis with liver disease or advanced renal insufficiency.	$
Alpha-Glucosidase Inhibitors: 1995 (acarbose, miglitol)	Inhibit absorption of carbohydrates from the small intestine	Bloating, flatulence Avoid with bowel diseases	$
Thiazolidinediones: 1999 (pioglitazone)	Insulin sensitizers, increase peripheral glucose uptake	Increase risk of congestive heart failure, weight gain, fracture risk, and bladder cancer	$
GLP-1 Agonists: 2005 (exenatide, liraglutide, dulaglutide lixisenatide + glargine, semaglutide)[c]	Increases gastric emptying time and stimulate glucose-dependent insulin secretion. Also decreases hepatic gluconeogenesis	Nausea/vomiting Pancreatitis Avoid with family history of medullary thyroid cancer	$$$$
DPP-4 Inhibitors: 2006 (sitagliptin, saxagliptin, linagliptin, alogliptin)[c]	Secretagogues: Stimulate B-cell insulin release in a meal dependent fashion	Alogliptin and saxagliptin assoc. with heart failure. Joint pains	$$$
SGLT-2 Inhibitors: 2013 (canagliflozin, dapagliflozin, empagliflozin, ertugliflozin)	Inhibit renal glucose reabsorption, thus increasing urinary glucose excretion	Increased urination, urinary tract infections and/yeast infections, dehydration and rarely ketoacidosis	$$$
GIP + GLP-1 Agonists: 2022 (tirzepatide)	Targets 2 incretin hormones—see GLP section.	See GLP section	$$$$

[a] Cost is calculated by average retail price of 1 month of therapy. http://www.goodrx.com. $ = $1-$99, $$ = $100-$299, $$$ = $300-$499, $$$$ = $500+.
[b] US Food and Drug Administration approval date. Dates are for the first agent in the class approved.
[c] DPP-4 and GLP-1 should not be used in combination with each other due to lack of benefit.[47]

Table 3
Food and Drug Administration-approved insulins by onset of action, concentrations, special features, and cost

Insulin	Concentration	Special Features	Cost
Rapid-acting Aspart Glulisine Lispro	U-100	Quick onset of action, duration of action 3–5 h	Pen = $$$ Vial = $$
Short-acting (Regular/R)	U-100	Duration of action 6–8 h	Vial = $
Intermediate- acting (Isophane/NPH) Regular	U-100 U-500	Duration of action 10–16 h Most concentrated Duration 6–10 h	Pen = $$ Vial = $$ Pen = $$$ Vial = $$
Long-acting Detemir Glargine Glargine (Toujeo)	U-100 U-100 U-300	Duration 21 h Duration 22–24 h. Duration 36 h	Pen/Vial = $$ Pen/Vial = $$ Pen = $$$$

Ultra-long- acting
Degludec
	U-100
	U-200
		Duration of action is 42 h.
		Does not need to be
		    injected at the same time
		    of the day
			Pen = $$
			Vial = $$
			U200 Pen = $$$$

Premixed
70% isophane/30% regular
70% aspart protamine &
    30% aspart
50% lispro protamine &
    50% lispro
75% lispro protamine &
    25% lispro
	U-100
	U-100
	U-100
	U-100
		Biphasic duration/peaks
		Biphasic
		Biphasic
		Biphasic
			Pen = $$
			Vial = $
			Pen = $
			Vial = $$
			Pen = $$$$
			Vial = $$$$
			Pen = $

Abbreviation: FDA, US food and drug administration.

confirming autoantibodies to islet cells, glutamic acid decarboxylase 65, insulin, tyrosine phosphatase IA-2 and IA-2beta, or zinc transporter 8 is diagnostic for type 1 diabetes.[20]

Levels of C-peptide, a byproduct on endogenous insulin production, are used to assess pancreatic beta-cell function and insulin secretion. A fasting C-peptide level of less than 0.6 ng per mL indicates insulin deficiency and is associated with type 1 diabetes.[22]

Prevalence

1.6 million adults aged 20 years or older—5.7% of all US adults with diagnosed diabetes—reported both having type 1 diabetes and using insulin.[16]

Table 4
Secondary causes of hypo and hyperglycemia

Hypoglycemia	Hyperglycemia
Hormone deficiencies	Endocrine disorders
Enzyme deficiencies	Medication induced
Low caloric intake	Pancreatic disease
Acquired liver diseases	Genetic syndromes
Hyperinsulism	Physiologic Stress
Metabolic deficiencies	

Age of presentation is bimodal: At 4 to 6 years of age and 10 to 14 years of age.[21]

Pathogenesis

Immune-mediated destruction of the pancreatic beta-cells. There is an inheritable susceptibility to T1DM with human leukocyte antigen (HLA) class 2 genes at 6p21 accounting for 30% to 50% of cases.[32]

Clinical Features

Body habitus is usually normal. Rapid onset of symptoms include polyphagia, polydipsia, polyuria, weight loss, and ketosis or diabetic ketoacidosis.

Evaluation and Diagnosis

The evaluation of Type I DM includes confirming an elevated glucose state and reduced insulin production. To differentiate between Type I and Type II DM, it is helpful to obtain a C-peptide and pancreatic antibodies.[20,21] C-peptide is a marker for endogenous insulin production. Therefore, a fasting C-peptide level of less than 0.6 ng per mL indicates insulin deficiency and is associated with type 1 diabetes.[22]

Acute and Chronic Complications

The chronic complications of DM1 mimic those for DM2. However, due to the early onset of DM1, chronic complications are seen at an earlier age. In a group of 11 to 17-year-old patients who had had type 1 diabetes for 2 to 5 years, early retinopathy was present in 9%, albuminuria was present in 3%, and there was a peripheral nerve abnormality in 16% when measured by thermal and vibration thresholds.[33]

The main acute complication of DM1 is diabetic ketoacidosis (DKA). Treatment principles for DKA include intravenous (IV) fluid resuscitation, IV insulin therapy with the addition of glucose depending on glucose levels, correction of acidosis, treatment of precipitating conditions, and correction of electrolytes.

Therapeutic Options

Insulin (see **Table 3**) which can be administered via an insulin pump in a basal/bolus fashion or injected in the traditional manner. Off-label use of metformin may lower insulin requirements.[34]

LATENT AUTOIMMUNE DIABETES IN ADULTS
Definition

A slow-progressing form of autoimmune diabetes affecting adults over 35 years of age. The Immunology for Diabetes Society has specified 3 criteria for the diagnosis of LADA.

1. Age greater than 35
2. Positive autoantibodies to islet beta cells
3. Insulin independence for at least the initial 6 months after diagnosis

Prevalence

Latent autoimmune diabetes in adults (LADA) is the most prevalent form of autoimmune diabetes as a whole.[35] In the multicentric "Action LADA" study from Europe, almost 10% of individuals with adult-onset DM had islet cell autoantibodies.

Pathogenesis

LADA is determined by genetic factors. As in T1DM, the risk for acquiring LADA is highest in carriers of certain HLA haplotypes. The HLA genes code for the major histocompatibility antigens which have important immunoregulatory functions, and therefore it is not surprising that LADA is caused by dysregulated immunity. However, the factors that precipitate autoimmunity have not been established.[35] The onset of symptom development, however, is more gradual than with DM1 since beta-cell destruction happens more slowly.

Clinical Features

A diagnostic screening tool with 3 criteria was used to identify LADA in diabetic patients older than 50 years of age.

1. A low or normal BMI.
2. A fasting blood glucose 270 mg/dL or higher, and HbA1C 10% or greater despite good compliance.
3. Loss of weight despite a diet constant in calorie content.

This tool is said to detect three-fourths of patients with LADA.[20]

C-peptide is cost-effective when used as the initial test to distinguish LADA from T2DM but has to be later confirmed with antibody testing.[36]

Acute and Chronic Complications

Early in the disease process, LADA behaves more like DM2, but as beta-cell destruction progresses, it starts resembling DM1. Long-term follow-up of patients with LADA reveals a lower risk in the first 9 years but a higher risk in later years for microvascular complications when compared to T2DM even after adjustment for several factors.[37]

Patients with LADA have as much carotid artery atherosclerosis as T1DM and T2DM despite a better vascular risk profile.[38]

GESTATIONAL DIABETES MELLITUS
Definition

Gestational diabetes is defined as diabetes mellitus that developed during pregnancy in a patient who was non-diabetic prior to pregnancy. Screening for gestational diabetes mellitus (GDM) is recommended at 24 to 28 weeks of gestation.[6] The glucose thresholds for diagnosis GDM are listed in **Box 1**.

Prevalence

GDM affects up to 1 in 11 pregnancies in the United States.[39]

Pathogenesis

As pregnancy progresses, a surge of local and placental hormones, including estrogen, progesterone, leptin, cortisol, placental lactogen, and placental growth hormone together promote a state of insulin resistance.[40] As a result, blood glucose is slightly elevated, and this glucose is readily transported across the placenta to fuel the growth of the fetus. This mild state of insulin resistance also promotes endogenous glucose production and the breakdown of fat stores, resulting in a further increase in blood glucose and free fatty acid (FFA) concentrations.[41]

Risk factors for developing GDM include genetic susceptibility, inactivity, increased BMI, and advanced maternal age.

> **Box 1**
> **Glucose thresholds for the diagnosis of gestational diabetes mellitus on different tolerance tests**
>
> *One-step method* = 75-g oral glucose tolerance test with measurements after 1 and 2 hours. For diagnosis of GDM, it requires only 1 abnormal result.
>
> Fasting 92 mg/dL
>
> 1-hour 180 mg/dL
>
> 2-hour 153 mg/dL
>
> *2-step method* = 50-g oral glucose tolerance test with measurement after an hour.
>
> If 1-hour glucose ≥ 135, conduct a diagnostic 100-g glucose tolerance test. The Carpenter-Coustan thresholds are as follows:
>
> Fasting 95 mg/dL
>
> 1-hour 180 mg/dL
>
> 2-hour 155 mg/dL
>
> 3-hour 140 mg/dL
>
> Self-monitoring levels (Glycemic targets during pregnancy are under these levels)
>
> Fasting 95 mg/dL
>
> 1-hour post prandial 140 mg/dL
>
> 2-hour post prandial 120 mg/dL
>
> *Information from* Refs.[39,44,56]

Acute and Chronic Complications

GDM increases the rates of C-sections, fetal macrosomia, shoulder dystocia, neonatal hypoglycemia, neonatal respiratory distress, and maternal hypertension.

Post-delivery, glucose levels typically normalize. However, the risk of developing overt diabetes within 25 years is 10 times higher in patients with a history of GDM compared with those who do not.[42]

Therapeutic Options

Lifestyle modification is the first-line intervention involving pre-pregnancy weight loss, and moderate exercise and dietary measures during pregnancy. A Cochrane review noted a reduction in cesarean delivery rate with the dietary approaches to stop hypertension diet in 2 trials with 86 patients.[43]

When medicines are necessary, the American College of Obstetricians and Gynecologists and the ADA primarily recommend insulin due to its long-standing safety profile, effectiveness, and inability to cross the placenta.[44] Metformin and glyburide can also be used, although glyburide has more adverse side effects.

MATURITY-ONSET DIABETES OF THE YOUNG
Introduction

Maturity-onset diabetes of the young (MODY) is a hereditary form of diabetes mellitus caused by impaired insulin secretion due to genetic mutations. It is a rare condition, accounting for approximately 1% of diabetes cases. MODY should be suspected in any non-obese patient diagnosed with diabetes mellitus before the age of 25 to 30 year old.[45] Although MODY can be divided into 14 subtypes, this article will focus on subtypes 1 to 3, as they account for 95% of all cases.

Pathogenesis

MODY 1 and 3 are caused by mutations in transcription factors which result in impaired insulin secretion from defective beta-cell signaling in response to glucose.[46]

MODY2 is caused by mutations in the GCK gene, resulting in a higher glucose set point for insulin secretion.[46]

Clinical Features

MODY should be considered in non-obese patients who have diabetes that was diagnosed at a young age, preserved pancreatic beta-cell function, lack of pancreatic beta-cell autoimmunity, and a strong family history of diabetes.[13] MODY patients display a lack of response to metformin. However, they are very responsive to sulfonylureas and insulin. Sulfonylureas push insulin out of the beta-cells in a non-glucose-dependent fashion; therefore, the signaling defect of MODY is overcome.

Evaluation and Diagnosis

MODY is frequently misdiagnosed as Type I DM or Type II DM. The age (young) and BMI (non-obese) of the patient are key clinical features that can help identify MODY. Laboratory evaluation involves obtaining an A1C, C-peptide level, and pancreatic autoantibodies. In MODY, the A1C is *greater than* 6.5%, the C-peptide level is low or low-normal, and autoantibodies are negative.[46]

Acute and Chronic Complications

Complications are dependent on the subtype of MODY> MODY 1 and 3 have the typical microvascular and macrovascular complications from suboptimal glycemic control while MODY2 is rarely associated with vascular complications.[47]

Therapeutic Options

Low-carbohydrate diet is beneficial with MODY 1 and 3 given the glucose intolerance and defective signaling. Sulfonylureas are the standard treatment for MODY and should be started at one-fourth of the typical starting dose to avoid hypoglycemia, then slowly titrated to achieve optimal glycemic control.[47] Insulin and other oral hypoglycemic agents are options for treatment of MODY when sulfonylureas fail to reach target A1C, are not tolerated, or are contraindicated.[47]

HYPOGLYCEMIA
Underproduction of Glucose

Hormone deficiencies
Hypothyroidism: Hypothyroid patients have relative adrenal insufficiency, even if they are not associated with primary adrenal failure. There is a blunted hypothalamic-pituitary-adrenal response to hypoglycemia in hypothyroid persons.[48]

Pituitary and Adrenal Disorders: Low levels of cortisol, growth hormone, glucagon, and epinephrine can also lead to hypoglycemia.

Addison disease: An acquired primary adrenal insufficiency. Autoimmune destruction of the adrenal glands is the most common cause of Addison disease.[49]

The adrenal glands make cortisol and aldosterone. A deficiency in these hormones leads to electrolyte abnormalities, hypoglycemia, and may ultimately produce an adrenal crisis.

Enzyme deficiencies
Phosphoenolpyruvate carboxykinase (PEPCK) deficiency is a disorder of carbohydrate metabolism. Cytosolic phosphoenolpyruvate carboxykinase (PEPCK) deficiency (MIM

261680, EC 4.1.1.32, encoded by PCK1) is a rare disorder of gluconeogenesis presenting with recurrent hypoglycemia, hepatic dysfunction, and lactic acidosis.[50]

Galactosemia: Galactosemia is an inborn disorder of carbohydrate metabolism characterized by the inability to metabolize galactose, a sugar contained in milk (the main source of nourishment for infants), and convert it into glucose, the sugar used by the body as the primary source of energy. Galactosemia is an autosomal recessive genetic disease that can be diagnosed at birth, even in the absence of symptoms, with newborn screening by assessing the level of galactose and the galactose-1-phosphate uridyltransferase (GALT) enzyme activity, as GALT defect constitutes the most frequent cause of galactosemia.[51]

Low caloric intake/malnutrition

Resulting from inadequate caloric intake, causing glycogen stores (which the body uses to create glucose) to become used up.

Acquired liver diseases

After a meal, there is a rise in blood glucose levels, which raises insulin secretion from the pancreas simultaneously. Insulin causes glucose to deposit in the liver as glycogen; then, during the next few hours, when blood glucose concentration falls, the liver releases glucose back into the blood, decreasing fluctuations.[52]

Clinical significance: During severe liver disease, it is impossible to maintain blood glucose concentration.[52]

Overconsumption of Glucose

Hyperinsulism

Can be due to medications such as exogenous insulin or sulfonylureas.

Endogenous causes include *Insulinomas.* Insulinomas primarily cause hypoglycemia in the fasting state, but may cause symptoms in the postprandial period as well. The incidence is 1/250,000 patient-years. Less than 10% are malignant, multiple, or present in patients with the multiple endocrine neoplasia type 1 (MEN-1) syndrome.[53]

Metabolic deficiencies

Fatty Acid Oxidation Disorders may lead to hypoketotic hypoglycemia.

Medium-chain acyl-CoA dehydrogenase deficiency. Affected patients are unable to synthesize ketone bodies for energy during times of fasting or acute stress; therefore, will present in metabolic crisis due to hypoketotic hypoglycemia. Although widespread use of newborn screens has decreased the acute crisis, these patients continue to present to the emergency department.[54]

Carnitine Transport Disorders. Carnitine is essential for the transfer of long-chain fatty acids across the inner mitochondrial membrane for subsequent β-oxidation. It can be synthesized by the body or assumed with the diet from meat and dairy products. Defects in the OCTN2 carnitine transporter results in autosomal recessive primary carnitine deficiency characterized by decreased intracellular carnitine accumulation, increased losses of carnitine in the urine, and low serum carnitine levels.[55]

CLINICS CARE POINTS

- DM 2 is characterized by impaired target tissue response to insulin, causing hyperglycemia and compensatory hyperinsulinemia. Eventually, there is beta-cell dysfunction and uncompensated hyperglycemia.

- DM 1 and LADA are caused by autoimmune destruction of the pancreatic beta-cells.
- MODY 1 and 3 result from defective beta-cell signaling in response to glucose which leads to decreased insulin secretion
- Acute blood loss and hemoglobinopathies are conditions which can alter A1C results.
- Secondary hyperglycemia can result from various endocrine disorders, medications, pancreatic disease, genetic syndromes, and physiologic stress
- Hypoglycemic causes can be separated into 2 major categories: 1) Underproduction of glucose due to hormone and enzyme deficiencies, liver disease, or malnutrition. 2) Overconsumption of glucose due to hyperinsulinism or metabolic deficiencies.

DISCLOSURE

The author has nothing to disclose.

REFERENCES

1. American Diabetic Association. Good to know: all about insulin resistance. Clin Diabetes 2018;36(3):263–4.
2. Huang Paul L. A comprehensive definition for metabolic syndrome. Disease models and mechanisms 2009;2(5–6):231–7.
3. Freeman AM, Acevedo LA, Pennings N. Insulin resistance. Treasure Island (FL): StatPearls Publishing; 2023.
4. Nasir NM, Thevarajah M, Yean CY. Hemoglobin variants detected by hemoglobin A1C analysis and the effects of HgbA1C measurements. Int J Diabetes Dev Ctries 2010;30(2):86–90.
5. Lapolla A, Mosca A, Fedele D. The general use of glycated hemoglobin for the diagnosis of diabetes and the other categories of glucose intolerance: still a long way to go. Nutr Metabol Cardiovasc Dis 2011;21(7):467–75.
6. Ferrau F, Albani A, Ciresi A, et al. Diabetes secondary to acromegaly: physiopathology, clinical features and effects of treatment. Front Endocrinol 2018;9:358.
7. Ray S, Ghosh S. Thyroid disorders and diabetes mellitus: double trouble. J Diabetes Res Ther 2016;2:1–7.
8. Pivonello R, De Leo M, Vitale P, et al. Pathophysiology of diabetes mellitus in Cushing's syndrome. Neuroendocrinology 2010;92(Suppl 1):77–81.
9. Wiesner TD, Blüher M, Windgassen M. Improvement of insulin sensitivity after adrenalectomy in patients with pheochromocytoma. J Clin Endocrinol Metab 2003;88:3632–6.
10. Holt R. Association between antipsychotic medication use and diabetes. Curr Diabetes Rep 2019;19(10):96.
11. Fonseca A, Carvalho E, Eriksson J, et al. Calcineurin is an important factor involved in human adipocytes. Mol Cell Biochem 2018;445(1):157–68.
12. Kaufman M, Simionatto C. A review of protease inhibitor-induced hyperglycemia. Pharmacotherapy 2012. https://doi.org/10.1592/phco.19.1.114.30514.
13. Magnisio jr CH, Spencer J. Insulin receptor antibodies and insulin resistance. Southern Med J 1999;92(7):717–9.
14. Mouri M, Barireddy M. Hyperglycemia. Treasure Island (FL). StatPearls Publishing; 2023.
15. American Diabetic Association. Standards of medical care in diabetes. Clin Diabetes 2020;38(1):10–38.

16. Centers for Disease Control and Prevention. National Diabetes Statistics Report Website. https://www.cdc.gov/diabetes/data/statistic-report/index.html. [Accessed 16 October 2023].

17. Echouffo-Tcheugui J, Selvin E. Pre-diabetes and what it means: The Epidemiological Evidence. Annu Rev Publ Health 2021;42:59–77.

18. Herman WH, Smith PJ, Thompson TJ, et al. A new and simple questionnaire to identify people at risk for undiagnosed diabetes. Diabetes Care 1995;18(3): 382–7.

19. American Diabetes Association. Standards of medical care. Diabetes Care 2020; 43(Supplement 1):S1–212.

20. Monge L, Bruno G, Pinach S, et al. A clinically orientated approach increases the efficiency of screening for latent autoimmune diabetes in adults (LADA) in a large clinic-based cohort of patients with diabetes onset over 50 years. Diabet Med 2004;21(5):456–9.

21. American Diabetes Association. Diagnosis and classification of diabetes mellitus. Diabetes Care 2013;36(suppl 1):S67–74.

22. Leighton E, Sainsbury CA, Jones GC. A practical review of C-peptide testing in diabetes. Diabetes Therapy 2017;8(3):475–87.

23. Brutsaert E., Diabetes mellitus. Merck Manual Professional Version, 2023, Merck and Co., Inc; Rahway, NJ, USA

24. Ebell MH, Grad R. Top 20 research studies of 2016 for primary care physicians. Am Fam Physician 2017;95(9):572–9.

25. Funtanilla V, Caliendo T, Hilas O. Continuous glucose monitoring: a review of available systems. Pharmacy and Therapeutics 2019;44(9):550–3.

26. Hemmingsen B, Gimenez-Perez G, Mauricio D, et al. Diet, physical activity or both for prevention or delay of type 2 diabetes mellitus and its associated complications in people at increased risk of developing type 2 diabetes mellitus. Cochrane Database Syst Rev 2017;(12):CD003054. https://doi.org/10.1002/14651858.CD003054.pub4.

27. Ilyas S, Al-Refai R, Maharjan R, et al. Bariatric surgery and type 2 diabetes mellitus: assessing factors leading to remission. a systematic review. Cureus 2020; 12(8):e9973.

28. Dahlen A, Dashi G, Maslov I, et al. Trends in antidiabetic drug discovery: FDA approved drugs, New Drugs in clinical trials and global sales. Front Pharmacol 2021;12:807548.

29. GoodRx, Available at: http://www.goodrx.com. Accessed February 22, 2024.

30. American Diabetes Association. Standards of medical care in diabetes-2017. Diabetes Care 2017;40(suppl 1):S1–135.

31. Garber AJ, Abrahamson MJ, Barzilay JI, et al. Consensus statement by the American Association of Clinical Endocrinologists and American College of Endocrinology on the comprehensive type 2 diabetes management algorithm-2016 executive summary. Endocr Pract 2016;22(1):84–113.

32. Felner EI, Klitz W, Ham M, et al. Genetic interaction among three genomic regions creates distinct contributions to early and late-onset type 1 diabetes mellitus. Pediatr Diabetes 2005;6(4):213–20.

33. Cho YH, Craig ME, Hing S, et al. Microvascular complications assessment in adolescents with 2- to 5-yr duration of type 1 diabetes from 1990 to (2006). Pediatr Diabetes 2011;(12):682–9.

34. Vella S, Buetow L, Royle P, et al. The use of metformin in type 1 diabetes: a systematic review of efficacy. Diabetologia 2010;53(5):809–20.

35. Laugesen E, Østergaard JA, Leslie RD. Danish diabetes academy workshop and workshop speakers. latent autoimmune diabetes of the adult: current knowledge and uncertainty. Diabet Med 2015;32(7):843–52.

36. Leighton E, Sainsbury CA, Jones GC. A practical review of C-peptide testing in diabetes. Diabetes Ther 2017;8(3):475–87.

37. Maddaloni E, Coleman RL, Agbaje O, et al. Time-varying risk of microvascular complications in latent autoimmune diabetes of adulthood compared with type 2 diabetes in adults: a post-hoc analysis of the UK Prospective Diabetes Study 30-year follow-up data (UKPDS 86). Lancet Diabetes Endocrinol 2020;8(3): 206–15.

38. Hernández M, López C, Real J, et al. Preclinical carotid atherosclerosis in patients with latent autoimmune diabetes in adults (LADA), type 2 diabetes and classical type 1 diabetes. Cardiovasc Diabetol 2017 28;16(1):94.

39. Pillay J, Donovan L, Guitard S, et al. Screening for gestational diabetes updated evidence report and systemic review for the US Preventive Services Task Force. JAMA 2021;326(6):539–62.

40. Catalano PM, Tyzbir ED, Roman NM, et al. Longitudinal changes in insulin release and insulin resistance in nonobese pregnant women. Am J Obstet Gynecol 1991; 165:1667–72.

41. Phelps RL, Metzger BE, Freinkel N. Carbohydrate metabolism in pregnancy: XVII. Diurnal profiles of plasma glucose, insulin, free fatty acids, triglycerides, cholesterol, and individual amino acids in late normal pregnancy. Am J Obstet Gynecol 1981;140:730–6.

42. Vounzoulaki E, Khunti K, Abner SC, et al. Progression to type 2 diabetes in women with a known history of gestational diabetes: systematic review and meta-analysis. BMJ 2020;369:m1361.

43. Han S, Middleton P, Shepherd E, et al. Different types of dietary advice for women with gestational diabetes mellitus. Cochrane Database Syst Rev 2017;(2): CD009275.

44. ACOG practice bulletin no. 190: gestational diabetes mellitus. Obstet Gynecol 2018;131(2):e49–64.

45. Nkonge KM, Nkonge DK, Nkonge TN. The epidemiology, molecular pathogenesis, diagnosis, and treatment of maturity-onset diabetes of the young (MODY). Clin Diabetes Endocrinology 2020;6(1):20.

46. Jang KM. Maturity-onset diabetes of the young update and perspectives on diagnosis and treatment. Yeungnam Univ J Med 2020;37(1):13–21.

47. Delvecchio M, Pastore C, Giordano P. Treatment options for MODY patients: a systematic review of the literature. Diabetes Ther 2020;11(8):1667–85.

48. Kamilaris TC, DeBold CR, Pavlou SN, et al. Effect of altered thyroid hormone levels on hypothalamic-pituitary-adrenal function. J Clin Endocrinol Metab 1987;65:994–9.

49. Michels AW, Eisenbarth GS. Immunologic endocrine disorders. J Allergy Clin Immunol 2010;125(2 Suppl 2):S226–37.

50. Becker J, Haas N, Valho S, et al. PEPCK Deficiency: Cause of Hypoglycemia-Induced Seizure and Death. Neuropediatrics 2021;52(5):398–402.

51. Succoio M, Sacchettini R, Alessandro R, et al. Galactosemia: biochemistry, molecular genetics, newborn screening, and treatment. Biomolecules 2022; 12(7):968.

52. Nakrani M, Wineland R, Anjum F. Physiology, glucose metabolism. St. Petersburg, FL, USA: Stat Pearls Publishing; 2023.

53. Cryer PE, Axelrod L, Grossman AB, et al. Evaluation and management of adult hypoglycemic disorders: an endocrine society clinical practice guideline. J Clin Endocrinol Metab 2009;94:709–28.
54. Andresen BS, Dobrowolski SF, O'Reilly L, et al. Medium-chain acyl-CoA dehydrogenase (MCAD) mutations identified by MS/MS-based prospective screening of newborns differ from those observed in patients with clinical symptoms: identification and characterization of a new, prevalent mutation that results in mild MCAD deficiency. Am J Hum Genet 2001;68(6):1408–18.
55. Longo N, Frigeni M, Pasquali M. Carnitine transport and fatty acid oxidation. Biochim Biophys Acta 2016;1863(10):2422–35.
56. Metzger BE, Gabbe SG, Persson B, et al. International Association of Diabetes and Pregnancy Study Groups Consensus Panel; International association of diabetes and pregnancy study groups recommendations on the diagnosis and classification of hyperglycemia in pregnancy. Diabetes Care 2010;33(3):676–82.

Calcium Disorders

Therese Anderson, MD*, Rebecca Bowie, MD,
Anna van Niekerk, DO

KEYWORDS

- Calcium disorders • Hypocalcemia • Hypercalcemia • Primary care

KEY POINTS

- Patients with hypercalcemia are often asymptomatic until levels reach greater than 12 mg/dL.
- The most common causes of elevated calcium levels are hyperparathyroidism and malignancy.
- The most common cause of hypocalcemia in primary care is vitamin D deficiency.
- Trousseau's sign is more specific than Chvostek's sign for hypocalcemia.
- Urgent treatment with intravenous calcium is indicated for severe hypocalcemia less than 7.5 mg/dL.

OVERVIEW OF PHYSIOLOGY

Calcium is the most abundant cation in the body. Over 99% of total body calcium is stored in our bones as hydroxyapatite.[1] Calcium (bound) is required for forming bones and teeth.

Serum total calcium, which is measured on a basic metabolic panel, has 3 forms: free, protein-bound, and anion-bound. Free (ionized) calcium is available for helping to form action potentials for muscle contraction. It is also necessary for cell division, secondary hemostasis (factor IV), and nerve conduction and is used as a second messenger for cell communication.[2]

Total serum calcium is broken down to (**Figs. 1** and **2**)

- 50% free (ionized), biologically active, and most clinically relevant form,
- 40% bound to protein, mostly albumin, but not used by tissues, and
- 10% bound to anions (phosphate, lactate, citrate), which is chelated (complexed) and can be absorbed by various tissues.

Serum calcium is regulated by parathyroid gland hormone (PTH), calcitonin (thyroid gland), and calcitriol (vitamin D) (**Table 1**). Calcium is absorbed in the intestine by

Department of Family Medicine, Mayo Clinic, 4500 San Pablo Road, Jacksonville, FL 32224, USA
* Corresponding author.
E-mail address: farmer.therese@mayo.edu

Prim Care Clin Office Pract 51 (2024) 391–403
https://doi.org/10.1016/j.pop.2024.03.004
primarycare.theclinics.com

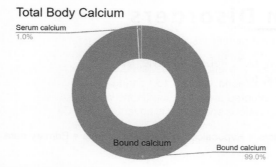

Fig. 1. Overview of total body calcium.

vitamin D. PTH mediates intestinal absorption, renal calcium retention, and bone resorption.

With a decline in serum calcium, PTH is secreted. PTH decreases renal calcium excretion and increases release of free calcium from bones. PTH will also increase renal conversion of 25-hydroxyvitamin D to calcitriol which can then increase intestinal calcium absorption.

With an increase in serum calcium, PTH is suppressed and calcitonin is released, leading to excretion of calcium by the kidneys. If there is no renal disease, the renal system can remove up to 400 mg of calcium per day.[3] Calcitonin will also stimulate calcium deposition into bones and inhibit intestinal calcium absorption.

CLINICS CARE POINTS

- Majority of total body calcium is bound in bones and teeth as calcium phosphate or hydroxyapatite.
- Free or ionized calcium is necessary for action potential for muscular contraction, cell division, and hemostasis and acts as a second messenger for cell communication.
- PTH is released in response to low serum calcium.
- PTH has action in the renal, gastrointestinal, and skeletal systems to increase serum calcium.
- Increased serum calcium stimulates release of thyroid calcitonin and inhibits PTH secretion.

HYPERCALCEMIA
Hypercalcemia Overview

Hypercalcemia is defined as a calcium level greater than the expected range, usually greater than 10.5 mg/dL depending on laboratory values. It is a disorder often found incidentally on blood work.[1] It is associated with very nonspecific symptoms and can affect the renal, gastrointestinal, neuromuscular, skeletal, and cardiovascular systems.

Clinical Features

Patients with incidentally found hypercalcemia are often asymptomatic. It is typically not until the calcium level reaches over 12 mg/dL that patients may display symptoms.

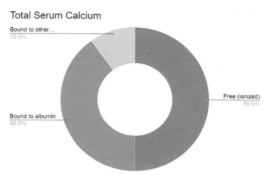

Fig. 2. Overview of total serum calcium.

A list of clinical manifestations by organ systems that can occur with hypercalcemia is given in **Table 2.**[4]

Etiologies

The most common causes of elevated calcium levels are hyperparathyroidism and malignancy.[5] Medications can often contribute to elevated calcium levels. Given that hyperparathyroidism is the most common cause of hypercalcemia, it is often categorized as PTH-mediated or non–PTH-mediated hypercalcemia.

PTH-mediated hypercalcemia[6]

- Primary hyperparathyroidism
  - It results in an increase in circulating PTH causing elevated calcium.
- Secondary hyperparathyroidism
  - It causes stimulation of the parathyroid glands, causing PTH release, typically from calcium homeostasis dysregulation.
- Tertiary hyperparathyroidism
  - This is usually related to chronic kidney disease (CKD) or vitamin D deficiency, causing PTH release due to a hypocalcemia state (excess phosphorous-binding calcium in CKD).

Non–PTH-mediated hypercalcemia

- Malignancy (solid tumors)

Table 1		
Regulation of serum calcium		
Organ System	**Low Serum Calcium**	**High Serum Calcium**
Endocrine system	Parathyroid glad releases PTH.	Thyroid gland (c-cells) releases calcitonin.
Gastrointestinal system	Vitamin D increases calcium absorption in the intestine.	Calcitonin inhibits calcium absorption in intestines.
Renal system	PTH increases renal calcium reabsorption and increases secretion of vitamin D3	Calcitonin inhibits renal reabsorption of calcium, increases urinary calcium excretion
Skeletal system	PTH stimulates osteoclasts leading to bone release of free calcium.	Calcitonin stimulates osteoblasts to deposit calcium in bones.

Abbreviation: PTH, parathyroid gland hormone.

Table 2
Manifestations of hypercalcemia

Organ System	Clinical Manifestation
Renal	Nephrolithiasis
	Polyuria
	Polydipsia
	Dehydration
Gastrointestinal	Constipation
	Nausea
	Abdominal pain
	Anorexia
Neuromuscular	Muscle weakness
	Confusion
	Fatigue
	Depression
Skeletal	Osteoporosis (fragility fractures)
	Subperiosteal resorption (bone cysts/tumors)
Cardiovascular	Hypertension
	Shortened QT interval
	Vascular calcification
Endocrine/Exocrine	Pancreatitis

- Excessive vitamin D
- Excessive exogenous calcium
- Medication-induced
- Granulomatous disease (eg, sarcoidosis)
- Endocrine disorders
  - Multiple endocrine neoplasia
  - Adrenal insufficiency
- Genetic
  - Familial hypercalciuric hypercalcemia
- Immobilization (eg, spinal cord injury or burn victim)
- Vitamin A toxicity
- Paget's disease

Diagnostic Evaluation

The first step in diagnosing hypercalcemia is often to repeat laboratory testing to ensure accuracy. If total calcium level reflects hypercalcemia, it should be classified as mild, moderate, or severe.[7]

- Mild is generally greater than 10 mg/dL to 12 mg/dL
- Moderate is generally 12 to 14 mg/dL
- Severe or hypercalcemic crisis is > 14 mg/dL

If the patient has clinical manifestations including unstable vital signs, electrocardiogram (EKG) changes, or mental status changes or the calcium level is > 12.5 mg/dL, this is considered a medical emergency.

If the patient is stable, and calcium level is mild or moderate, an outpatient workup may be appropriate. Once a full medication reconciliation has been completed, the outpatient workup for hypercalcemia is based on PTH function. Initial laboratory tests for hypercalcemia workup should include PTH, phosphorus, and vitamin D levels to determine etiology. Albumin and creatinine levels are recommended as well. An ionized calcium level is rarely helpful in an outpatient workup. A corrected albumin level may be helpful, and this can be determined by using the following formula:

Corrected calcium (mg/dL) = (4.0 per dL – [plasma albumin])3.08 + serum calcium mg/dL

A 24-hour urine collection can further classify hypercalcemia, particularly when the PTH level is normal or high. A low 24-hour urine calcium level may indicate abnormal kidney processing of calcium, like familial hypocalciuric hypercalcemia (FHH) in which there is a genetic defect in the calcium-sensing receptor (CaSR) of the kidney.[8] A normal or high urinary calcium level may indicate primary or tertiary hyperparathyroidism, as this is an appropriate response of the kidneys to excrete calcium in the urine with blood levels containing excessive amounts of calcium.

History should include a full medication reconciliation as many common medications are associated with hypercalcemia (**Box 1**).

MANAGEMENT OF HYPERCALCEMIA

Management is based on etiology of elevated calcium, severity of elevation, and symptomatology. Patients symptomatic with calcium greater than 12 mg/dL or asymptomatic with calcium greater than 14 mg/dL require prompt treatment with intravenous (IV) saline followed by calcium-lowering medications.

Mild hypercalcemia (asymptomatic and calcium <1 mg/dL above the upper limit of normal) requires adequate hydration, mobilization, and avoidance of nephrotoxic medications including anti-inflammatories.

For mild cases, recommend limiting dietary calcium to 1000 mg per day. It is also recommended to correct vitamin D deficiency to the goal range of 20 to 30 ng/mL. With mild hypercalcemia, consider medication side effects and discontinue the causative agent if possible.

FHH rarely leads to surgical intervention. Calcimimetics and calcilytics (CaSR antagonists) can be considered to improve disorders of the CaSR.[11,12]

Parathyroid Hormone–Dependent Causes

Primary hyperparathyroidism must lead to consideration for surgical intervention and assessment for surgical indications as written in **Table 3**.

Postmenopausal women with mild primary hyperparathyroidism may benefit from treatment with hormone replacement therapy (HRT).[13] HRT has little effect on serum calcium but can increase bone mineral density (BMD) and may ultimately stop patients from being surgical candidates.[14,15]

Box 1
Medications and supplements associated with hypercalcemia[9,10]

Calcium supplements

Vitamin D supplements

Recombinant PTH

Vitamin A analogs

Tamoxifen

Lithium

Thiazide diuretics

Table 3	
Treatment option pharmacokinetics	
Medication	**Time to Action**
Furosemide	6 h
Calcitonin	4–6 h
Bisphosphonates	24–48 h
Steroids	2–7 d
Denosumab	7–10 d

Parathyroid Hormone–Independent Causes

Malignancy hypercalcemia

Hypercalcemia of malignancy is primarily treated with bisphosphonates to inhibit osteoclast action and bone resorption. If unable to use bisphosphonates due to renal injury, consider denosumab.[16]

Bisphosphonates options include IV pamidronate and IV zoledronic acid. Hydrocortisone IV can also be used for hematologic malignancies after IV fluids. Steroids will inhibit vitamin D conversion to calcitriol and decrease the intestinal absorption of calcium. Mithramycin can block osteoclastic function but has a significant side effect profile to consider.

Vitamin-D intoxication and granulomatous disease

Steroids are the treatment of choice for excess vitamin D (calcitriol)–mediated hypercalcemia including granulomatous disease. Typical treatment includes IV hydrocortisone for 3 to 5 days followed by oral prednisone for 7 days.[14] Ketoconazole has a similar mechanism of action to steroids and can be used as well.[17]

HYPERCALCEMIC CRISIS

Hypercalcemic crisis (calcium>14, altered mental status, renal dysfunction, EKG changes) requires prompt IV saline and subsequent calcium-lowering medications like furosemide, calcitonin, and bisphosphonates.[9] The immediate goal is restoring intravascular volume and urinary calcium excretion. IV hydration is completed using normal saline to achieve a goal urine output of 200 mL/h.

Bisphosphonates or denosumab (if renal injury) and calcitonin can be used together based on time to action as shown in **Table 3**. During treatment, caution for overhydration is advised with any comorbid renal dysfunction or heart disease. Hemodialysis is the treatment of choice in patients with heart failure or renal insufficiency.[16,18,19]

Calcitonin has mild effects and is limited to a few days.

SURGICAL INTERVENTION

Indications for surgical intervention include patients with symptomatic primary hyperparathyroidism, age less than 50, elevated calcium greater than 1 mg/dL over normal, skeletal complications, increased risk for nephrolithiasis, and reduced renal function.[16] One in three patients with asymptomatic primary hyperparathyroidism will develop indications for surgery over 10 to 15 years (**Box 2**).

Surgical management with parathyroidectomy results in 95% cure rate. Known risks to surgical management include hypocalcemia and tetany. Hungry bone syndrome (significant hypocalcemia more than 4 days postoperatively) can occur with rapid

---

Box 2
Indications for parathyroid surgery

Indication for surgical intervention based on National Institutes of Health criteria
    Elevated calcium greater than 12 mg/dL
    History of life-threatening hypercalcemia
    Creatinine clearance reduced by 30% compared to age-matched normal
    Elevated 24-h urine calcium greater than 400 mg/d
    Nephrolithiasis
    Age less than 50
    Osteitis fibrosa cystica
    Bone mass greater than 2 standard deviations below control matched for age, gender, and ethnic group
    Neuromuscular complications: hyperreflexia, proximal weakness, atrophy

---

calcium into bones and may require IV calcium.[16] Patients may require calcium supplementation for up to 1 year.[11]

One year after surgery, patients can expect to have increased BMD, particularly in the spine.

CLINICS CARE POINTS

- Hungry bone syndrome is an important postoperative complication.

- Monitoring after surgical correction includes assessing BMD after surgery.

- Endocrinology should be involved with unclear underlying etiology hypercalcemia, pediatric-onset hypercalcemia, and if parathyroidectomy is warranted.

HYPOCALCEMIA

Hypocalcemia is a common electrolyte disorder. It is defined as corrected total serum calcium levels less than 8.5 mg/dL (<2.12 mml/L).[20] The most common cause of hypocalcemia in primary care is vitamin D deficiency,[21] though the following causes should also be considered:

- Chronic renal disease
- Medications
- Hypoparathyroidism
- Acute illness such as pancreatitis, rhabdomyolysis, or tumor lysis syndrome

Clinical Features

Hypocalcemia may be commonly diagnosed in an asymptomatic patient due to an incidental laboratory finding, as well as in a symptomatic patient.

The symptomatic patient may present with paresthesias, muscle twitching, or spasms, though neuromuscular symptoms and signs are usually limited to those patients with severe hypocalcemia. These may include spontaneous or provoked carpopedal spasm (Trousseau's sign) as well as facial nerve muscle spasm, provoked by percussion over the facial nerve at the level of the parotid gland (Chvostek's sign). Of the 2, Trousseau's sign is more specific for hypocalcemia, with positivity of 94% in hypocalcemic patients, as a larger portion of the general population have Chvostek's sign with normal calcium.[22]

Severe hypocalcemia (<7.5 mg/dL) can cause laryngospasm, seizure, myocardial dysfunction, and QT-interval prolongation, leading to sudden cardiac death. This may occur without preceding muscle cramping or paresthesias.[23]

Laboratory Assessment

Hypocalcemia should be confirmed with second measurement. In addition to obtaining serum calcium, serum albumin should also be obtained and calcium corrected for albumin levels, as 40% of calcium is protein-bound.[24] As with hypercalcemia, serum calcium should be corrected for albumin.[20] In patients with an acid-base disorder or critical illness, ionized calcium is preferred for the diagnosis of hypocalcemia.[24]

If the cause of hypocalcemia is not readily known, then the following laboratory values should be obtained:[20,25]

- PTH
- 25-hydroxyvitamin D
- Serum phosphate
- Magnesium
- Blood urea nitrogen
- Serum creatinine

Etiologies

Vitamin D deficiency

Vitamin D deficiency can occur in individuals with low ultraviolet light exposure, malabsorption (eg, celiac disease, bariatric surgery), or low dietary intake of vitamin D. Medications, such as anticonvulsants, are associated with hypocalcemia due to vitamin D deficiency.[26]

Hypoparathyroidism

Hypoparathyroidism is diagnosed by low or normal intact PTH, low serum corrected calcium, and normal 25-hydroxyvitamin D.[27,28] The most common cause of hypocalcemia due to PTH is surgical hypoparathyroidism.[27] Other causes of hypoparathyroidism can include autoimmune, metabolic, or malignant etiology.[20,27,28] Hypomagnesemia can also impair PTH secretion.[23] Genetic hypoparathyroidism is considered a rare cause of hypocalcemia, though it should be considered in the young adult with no other identifiable etiology.[20,25] Infiltrative diseases, such as hemochromatosis or Wilson disease, can result in insufficient PTH secretion.[20] PTH resistance, also known as pseudohypoparathyroidism, is another rare genetic cause of hypocalcemia, which results in PTH resistance (and thus elevated PTH), elevated phosphorus, and normal 25-hydroxyvitamin D level.[27,28] Patients with nonsurgical hypoparathyroidism may have presentations other than hypocalcemia, including cataracts, dental abnormalities, increased risk of infection, cardiovascular disease, and fractures.[28]

Chronic renal disease

In patients with chronic renal disease, hypocalcemia can result due to hyperphosphatemia and decreased 1alpha,25-dihydroxyvitamin D3 [$1,25(OH)_2D_3$] production, which may require supplementation with calcium as well as phosphate-binding agents.[23,29]

Medications

Box 3 highlights medications associated with hypocalcemia. It is particularly important to assess serum calcium and phosphate levels as well as 25-hydroxyvitamin D levels prior to initiation of bisphosphonate or denosumab therapy for osteoporosis.

> **Box 3**
> **Medications associated with hypocalcemia[20]**
>
> Loop diuretics
>
> Phosphate and magnesium supplementation
>
> Ethylenediaminetetraacetic acid
>
> Bisphosphonates
>
> Calcitonin
>
> Denosumab

Other etiologies

Acute illnesses such as rhabdomyolysis and tumor lysis syndrome can result in low ionized calcium.[20,23] Acute pancreatitis can result in saponification of calcium, resulting in hypocalcemia (and hypomagnesemia). Osteoblastic metastases, as seen in prostate and breast cancer, can cause hypocalcemia.[20,23] Hungry bone syndrome can result from a rapid shift of calcium into bones after parathyroidectomy for primary hyperparathyroidism.[20,23]

MANAGEMENT

Management is based on the chronicity and underlying cause of hypocalcemia. The goal of treatment is to resolve symptoms and increase serum calcium, vitamin D, and magnesium to normal ranges.[20] Urgent treatment with IV calcium is indicated for severe hypocalcemia less than 7.5 mg/dL. This requires monitoring with EKG.

Acute Hypocalcemia

Serum calcium below 1.9 mmol/L or ionized calcium less than 1 mmol/L below range or symptomatic hypocalcemia is treated with IV calcium salts. Blood calcium will need to be regularly monitored until a stable regimen is found. Dosing of calcium is dependent on the severity of deficiency. Increasing severe deficiency helps to prevent prolonged cardiac muscle depolarization and stabilize membrane potential.[2]

IV calcium gluconate has a lower risk of tissue necrosis if extravasated and is used more commonly. Both calcium gluconate and chloride, if being bolused, require EKG monitoring.

Chronic Hypocalcemia

For patients with long-standing hypocalcemia, it is important to have sufficient (1 g daily divided) dietary calcium and consider removing any medications that may limit calcium absorption. If dietary intake is insufficient, oral supplementation is recommended. Calcium is given 1 to 3 g total daily, divided 3 times daily and taken with meals. The intestine absorbs 200 to 400 mg of supplemented calcium.[2] No more than 500 mg per dose is recommended to maximize absorption. Long-term calcium supplementation can have significant gastrointestinal side effects including constipation, diarrhea, and abdominal pain.[3] For mild or chronic hypocalcemia, ensure vitamin D supplementation to achieve goal. It is also important to correct for concomitant hypomagnesemia.

Calcium supplementation can increase the risk for formation of calcium oxalate renal stones. Adequate dietary calcium may reduce the absorption of oxalate and

Table 4 Foods high in calcium[32]	
High Calcium Foods	**Calcium (mg) per Serving**
Tofu (raw)	434 (½ cup)
Yogurt, plain, low-fat	415 (8oz)
Sardines, canned	351 (3.75oz)
Cheddar cheese	303 (1.5oz)
Milk (dairy)	300 (8oz)
Bok choy	79 (½ cup)
Fig (dried)	61 ($\frac{1}{4}$ cup)
Orange	60 (1 medium)
Kale (cooked)	47 (1.2 cups)

the risk of stone formation.[30,31] Calcium is most bioavailable in foods mentioned in **Table 4**.[32]

The most common oral calcium supplements are calcium citrate and calcium carbonate. Calcium citrate is absorbed independent of food intake and should be used in patients using acid blockers.[33] Calcium carbonate is recommended to take during meals to ensure absorption. This formulation may interfere with absorption of other medications including levothyroxine.[33] Calcium carbonate is also more associated with constipation, flatulence, and bloating.[34]

While adequate supplementation is primary, it is important to also avoid hypercalciuria. Increased hypercalciuria increases the risk of extraskeletal calcifications and nephrolithiasis. Thiazide diuretics increase calcium reabsorption with a goal of urine calcium of 300 mg daily. Thiazide starting dose is 12.5 mg daily and is used up to 25 mg daily.

Hypoparathyroidism

After treatment with calcium and vitamin D or if unresponsive to treatment with calcitriol, recombinant human PTH can also be administered as a long-term treatment with known side effects of hypercalciuria.[35,36] Hypoparathyroidism with undetectable PTH or renal failure requires treatment with calcitriol.

CLINICS CARE POINTS

- The goal of therapy is serum calcium at or just below normal range without hypercalciuria.
- Calcium, vitamin D, and thiazide diuretics are the mainstays of the treatment.
- Calcitriol is indicated with renal failure or hypoparathyroidism with undetectable PTH.
- Hypercalciuria will limit therapy.
- Thiazide diuretics decrease urinary calcium excretion.
- Treat co-occurring hypomagnesemia.
- Treat co-occurring hyperphosphatemia; reduce intake of phosphate binders
- If hypocalcemia persists after treatment with calcitriol and calcium, it may require recombinant human PTH.

DISCLOSURE

The authors declare that they have no relevant or material financial or personal interests to disclose.

REFERENCES

1. Carroll Mary F, David S, Schade MD. A practical approach to hypercalcemia. Am Fam Physician 2003;67(9):1959–66.
2. Yu E, Sharma S. Physiology, calcium. In: StatPearls [Internet]. Treasure Island (FL): StatPearls Publishing; 2023. Available at: https://www.ncbi.nlm.nih.gov/books/NBK482128/.
3. Smith LM, Gallagher JC. Reference range for 24-h urine calcium, calcium/creatinine ratio, and correlations with calcium absorption and serum vitamin D metabolites in normal women. Osteoporos Int 2021;32(3):539–47.
4. Shane E. Hypercalcemia: pathogenesis, clinical manifestations, differential diagnosis, and management. In: Favus MJ, editor. Primer on the metabolic bone diseases and disorders of mineral metabolism. 4th edition. Philadelphia: Lippincott: Williams & Wilkins; 1999. p. 183–7.
5. Carrick AI, Costner HB. Rapid fire: hypercalcemia. Emerg Med Clin North Am 2018;36(3):549–55.
6. Fraser WD. Hyperparathyroidism. Lancet 2009;374(9684):145–58.
7. El-Hajj Fuleihan G, Clines GA, Hu MI, et al. Treatment of hypercalcemia of malignancy in adults: an endocrine society clinical practice guideline. J Clin Endocrinol Metabol 2023;108(3):507–28.
8. Kos CH, Karaplis AC, Peng JB, et al. The calcium-sensing receptor is required for normal calcium homeostasis independent of parathyroid hormone. J Clin Invest 2003;111(7):1021–8.
9. Lecoq AL, Livrozet M, Blanchard A, et al. Drug-related hypercalcemia. Endocrinol Metab Clin North Am 2021;50(4):743–52.
10. Seymour JF, Gagel RF. Calcitriol: the major humoral mediator of hypercalcemia in Hodgkin's Disease and Non-Hodgkin's Lymphomas. Blood 1993;82(5):1383–94. ISSN 0006-4971.
11. Afzal M, Kathuria P. Familial hypocalciuric hypercalcemia. In: StatPearls [Internet]. Treasure Island (FL): StatPearls Publishing; 2023. Available at: https://www.ncbi.nlm.nih.gov/books/NBK459190/.
12. Cartwright C, Anastasopoulou C. Hungry bone syndrome. In: StatPearls [Internet]. Treasure Island (FL): StatPearls Publishing; 2023. Available at: https://www.ncbi.nlm.nih.gov/books/NBK549880/.
13. Orr-Walker BJ, Evans MC, Clearwater JM, et al. Effects of hormone replacement therapy on bone mineral density in postmenopausal women with primary hyperparathyroidism: four-year follow-up and comparison with healthy postmenopausal women. Arch Intern Med 2000;160:2161–6.
14. Grey AB, Stapleton JP, Evans MC, et al. Effect of hormone replacement therapy on bone mineral density in postmenopausal women with mild primary hyperparathyroidism. A randomized, controlled trial. Ann Intern Med 1996;125(5):360–8. PMID: 8702086.
15. Sternlicht H, Glezerman IG. Hypercalcemia of malignancy and new treatment options. Therapeut Clin Risk Manag 2015;11:1779–88. PMID: 26675713; PMCID: PMC4675637.

16. Wang Y, Ladie DE. Parathyroidectomy. In: StatPearls [Internet]. Treasure Island (FL): StatPearls Publishing; 2023. Available at: https://www.ncbi.nlm.nih.gov/books/NBK563274/.

17. Bia MJ, Insogna K. Treatment of sarcoidosis-associated hypercalcemia with ketoconazole. Am J Kidney Dis 1991;18(6):702–5. PMID: 1962657.

18. Kaiser W, Biesenbach G, Kramar R, et al. Calcium free hemodialysis: an effective therapy in hypercalcemic crisis–report of 4 cases. Intensive Care Med 1989; 15(7):471–4. PMID: 2600293.

19. Fitzpatrick LA, Bilezikian JP. Acute primary hyperparathyroidism. Am J Med 1987; 82(2):275–82. PMID: 3812520.

20. Pepe J, Colangelo L, Biamonte F, et al. Diagnosis and management of hypocalcemia. Endocrine 2020;69(3):485–95. https://doi.org/10.1007/s12020-020-02324-2.

21. Holick MF. Vitamin D deficiency. N Engl J Med 2007;357(3):266–81. https://doi.org/10.1056/NEJMra070553.

22. Urbano FL. Signs of hypocalcemia: Chvostek's and Trousseau's. Hosp Physician 2000;36:43–5.

23. Bushinsky DA, Monk RD. Electrolyte quintet: Calcium [published correction appears in Lancet 2002 Jan 19;359(9302):266]. Lancet 1998;352(9124):306–11. https://doi.org/10.1016/s0140-6736(97)12331-5.

24. Slomp J, van der Voort PH, Gerritsen RT, et al. Albumin-adjusted calcium is not suitable for diagnosis of hyper- and hypocalcemia in the critically ill. Crit Care Med 2003;31(5):1389–93. https://doi.org/10.1097/01.CCM.0000063044.55669.3C.

25. Cooper MS, Gittoes NJL. Diagnosis and management of hypocalcaemia. BMJ 2008;336:1298.

26. Hahn TJ, Hendin BA, Scharp CR, et al. Effect of chronic anticonvulsant therapy on serum 25-hydroxycalciferol levels in adults. N Engl J Med 1972;287(18): 900–4. https://doi.org/10.1056/NEJM197211022871803.

27. Sell J, Ramirez S, Partin M. Parathyroid disorders. Am Fam Physician 2022; 105(3):289–98.

28. Gafni RI, Collins MT. Hypoparathyroidism. N Engl J Med 2019;380(18):1738–47. https://doi.org/10.1056/NEJMcp1800213.

29. Marx SJ. Hyperparathyroid and hypoparathyroid disorders [published correction appears in N Engl J Med 2001 Jan 18;344(3):240] [published correction appears in N Engl J Med 2001 Mar 1;344(9):696]. N Engl J Med 2000;343(25):1863–75. https://doi.org/10.1056/NEJM200012213432508.

30. Sorensen MD, Eisner BH, Stone KL, et al. Impact of calcium intake and intestinal calcium absorption on kidney stones in older women: the study of osteoporotic fractures. J Urol 2012;187(4):1287–92.

31. Bailey RL, Dodd KW, Goldman JA, et al. Estimation of total usual calcium and vitamin D intakes in the United States. J Nutr 2010;140(4):817–22.

32. Shkembi B, Huppertz T. Calcium absorption from food products: food matrix effects. Nutrients 2021;14(1):180. PMID: 35011055; PMCID: PMC8746734.

33. Straub DA. Calcium supplementation in clinical practice: a review of forms, doses, and indications. Nutr Clin Pract 2007;22(3):286–96.

34. Li K, Wang XF, Li DY, et al. The good, the bad, and the ugly of calcium supplementation: a review of calcium intake on human health. Clin Interv Aging 2018; 13:2443–52. PMID: 30568435; PMCID: PMC6276611.

35. Mannstadt M, Clarke BL, Vokes T, et al. Efficacy and safety of recombinant human parathyroid hormone (1-84) in hypoparathyroidism (REPLACE): a double-blind, placebo-controlled, randomised, phase 3 study [published correction appears in Lancet Diabetes Endocrinol. 2014 Jan;2(1):e3. Dosage error in article text]. Lancet

Diabetes Endocrinol 2013;1(4):275–83. https://doi.org/10.1016/S2213-8587(13) 70106-2.

36. Gafni RI, Guthrie LC, Kelly MH, et al. Transient increased calcium and calcitriol requirements after discontinuation of human synthetic parathyroid hormone 1-34 (hPTH 1-34) replacement therapy in hypoparathyroidism. J Bone Miner Res 2015;30(11):2112–8. https://doi.org/10.1002/jbmr.2555.

Thyroid Disorders

Gauri Dhir, MD[a], Vasudha Jain, MD[b,*], Andrew Merritt, MD[c]

KEYWORDS

- Hypothyroidism • Hyperthyroidism • Sick euthyroid • Grave's disease
- Hashimoto's disease • Subclinical thyroid disease • Myxedema coma

KEY POINTS

- Subclinical thyroid disease is defined by the presence of a disease without clinical symptoms usually when thyrotropin-releasing hormone (TSH) is greater than or less than the reference range with normal levels of free thyroxine and triiodothyronine concentrations.
- Subclinical hypothyroidism has been associated with increased risk of heart failure, particularly when TSH levels are above 10 mIU/L.
- Treatment of subclinical hypothyroidism is usually recommended when TSH is above 10 mIU/L.
- Treatment of subclinical hyperthyroidism is usually recommended when TSH is suppressed less than 0.1 mIU/L.
- Most common cause of hypothyroidism in an iodine-rich country is autoimmune thyroiditis.

GENERAL PRINCIPLES OF THYROID ENDOCRINOLOGY

The thyroid gland is located on the anterior neck and is an endocrine gland that affects several organ systems and their functions including cardiac output, thermoregulation, oxygen delivery to tissues, fetal growth, stimulating the nervous system, and playing a part in reproductive health.[1] Thyrotropin-releasing hormone is produced in the hypothalamus and stimulates the pituitary to release thyroid-stimulating hormone (TSH). The TSH is then responsible for stimulating the thyroid gland to make iodothyronines (free thyroxine [T4], triiodothyronine [T3], and reverse T3). Since TSH is released from the pituitary and then stimulates the thyroid gland to produce iodothyronines, there is an inverse correlation between TSH and the iodothyronines. T4 is converted peripherally into T3, and measurement of both iodothyronines is typically used for evaluation of thyroid function.

[a] Department of Endocrinology, Tidelands Health System, 4040 Highway 17 Bypass, Suite 306, Murrells Inlet, SC 29576, USA; [b] Department of Family Medicine, Tidelands Health MUSC Family Medicine Residency, 4320 Holmestown Road, Myrtle Beach, SC 29577, USA; [c] Department of Family Medicine, Tidelands Health Family Medicine Residency Program, 4320 Holmestown Road, Myrtle Beach, SC 29588, USA
* Corresponding author.
E-mail address: vjain@tidelandshealth.org

Prim Care Clin Office Pract 51 (2024) 405–415
https://doi.org/10.1016/j.pop.2024.04.001
0095-4543/24/© 2024 Elsevier Inc. All rights reserved.

HYPOTHYROIDISM
Introduction

Hypothyroidism is a common condition associated with thyroid hormone deficiency and an underactive thyroid. The most common signs and symptoms of hypothyroidism include fatigue, weight gain, depression, constipation, and skin changes. In the elderly, hypothyroidism can manifest as memory loss.

Worldwide, nutritional iodine deficiency is the most common cause of hypothyroidism.[2] Hypothyroidism can further be classified as primary, central (includes secondary and tertiary), and peripheral hypothyroidism (**Table 1**). Primary hypothyroidism is secondary to the destruction of the thyroid gland. Central hypothyroidism is due to pituitary or hypothalamic causes with a normal thyroid gland. Peripheral hypothyroidism is a consumptive hypothyroidism with overexpression of the deiodinase 3 enzyme in tumor tissues which inactivates thyroid hormone.[4]

In iodine-rich areas, chronic autoimmune thyroiditis (AITD), that is, Hashimoto's disease, is the most common cause of hypothyroidism. AITD is more common in women and in individuals with other autoimmune diseases or a family history of AITD. Other common causes of hypothyroidism include radiation therapy and the removal of the thyroid gland.[3,4] Controversy exists amongst different societies about screening for hypothyroidism in healthy adults with some societies recommending screening for hypothyroidism based on age and/or gender, while the US Preventive Services Task Force notes "insufficient evidence to make a screening recommendation."[5,6]

Presentation

Patients can present with a variety of signs and symptoms from hypothyroidism, but commonly include fatigue, weight gain, depression, constipation, skin changes, and can also include cold intolerance, menometrorrhagia, and sexual dysfunction.

Evaluation

The initial and most sensitive screening test of choice in the evaluation of hypothyroidism is a TSH assay. With an abnormal TSH assay, a reflex to free T4 test should be performed. Primary and peripheral hypothyroidism are characterized by high TSH and low thyroid hormone levels.[4] Central hypothyroidism, on the other hand, is characterized by a low to normal TSH and free T4.[4,7] If central hypothyroidism is suspected, a T4 test should be ordered with the TSH as part of the initial screening.[8]

Once the diagnosis of primary hypothyroidism is made, if necessary, further evaluation for the underlying etiology can be performed. However, in iodine-sufficient areas where AITD is the most likely cause, further evaluation is typically not necessary. If further evaluation is warranted, the clinician can measure thyroid peroxidase antibodies which would be elevated with AITD.[7]

Table 1
Hypothyroidism classifications[3]

Primary	Central (Secondary and Tertiary)	Peripheral
Autoimmune thyroiditis	Pituitary cause	Vascular tumor
Iodine deficiency	Hypothalamic cause	Fibrotic tumor
Acquired hypothyroidism	Drugs	Gastric stromal tumor
Transient thyroiditis		
Thyroid gland infiltration		
Genetic causes		

Treatment

The goal of treatment for hypothyroidism is a euthyroid state defined as a normal TSH between 0.45 and 4.12.[6] In those ≥70 years old, American Thyroid Association treatment goals are more liberal between 4 and 6.[8] In the elderly, thyroid dysfunction is associated with higher mortality and morbidity especially in the hospital setting.[9]

Levothyroxine remains the mainstay of hypothyroidism treatment with a usual starting dose for overt hypothyroidism of 1.6 mcg/kg/day, but this can be adjusted for age and comorbidities. For young asymptomatic patients, the weight-based starting dose of levothyroxine is reasonable, regardless of TSH and free T4 levels.[9] For patients with coronary artery disease and elderly patients, however, a starting dose is typically 12.5 to 25 mcg/day and titrated up slowly based on symptoms.[9,10] After treatment initiation, TSH should be retested in 4 to 8 weeks until a euthyroid state is achieved. Symptoms may begin to improve within 2 to 3 weeks, but a steady-state TSH concentration might not be achieved until 6 weeks.[11] For stable treated hypothyroidism, there is no consensus, but a TSH every 6 months is reasonable. For central hypothyroidism the free T4 level, not TSH, should guide the treatment of hypothyroidism.[8]

Levothyroxine should be taken on an empty stomach in the morning 30 to 60 - minutes before food or other medications. Medications known to impact effective levothyroxine levels include estrogen, sertraline, phenobarbital, carbamazepine, phenytoin, rifampicin, calcium carbonate, iron, proton pump inhibitors, warfarin, and sucralfate.[12,13]

HYPERTHYROIDISM
Introduction

To review, TSH is secreted by the pituitary and stimulates the thyroid gland to increase production of iodothyronines (free T4 and T3).[1] Hyperthyroidism is defined as an overactive thyroid gland resulting in suppressed TSH with high free T4 levels. Common etiologies include Grave's disease, toxic multinodular goiter, toxic adenoma, and painless thyroiditis.[14–16] Secondary hyperthyroidism is rare, and is usually caused by TSH-producing pituitary adenomas.

Etiologies of Thyrotoxicosis

Primary hyperthyroidism, or innate hyperactivity of the thyroid gland, is the most common cause of hyperthyroidism. As these etiologies are forms of a hyperfunctioning gland, each will show increased uptake on radioactive iodine (RAI) scan.[15]

The differential diagnosis for thyrotoxicosis includes metastatic follicular thyroid carcinoma or trophoblastic tumors. Other causes of thyrotoxicosis include consumption of exogenous thyroid hormone, where someone takes thyroid hormone to create a hyperthyroid state, and thyroiditis, which is related to inflammation of the thyroid gland. Thyroiditis may be related to or precipitated by viral illness, a post-partum state (up to 1 year), or medications, including iodine and amiodarone.[15] Although rare, ectopic pregnancy is another cause of hyperthyroidism and thyrotoxicosis. In this condition, the elevated levels of human chorionic gonadotropin (hCG), which is chemically analogous to TSH, stimulates excessive thyroid hormone production.[16]

Clinical Manifestations

Thyrotoxicosis and hyperthyroidism should be considered in the differential diagnosis for patients who present with signs and symptoms consistent with a hyperadrenergic or hypermetabolic state such as weight loss, heat intolerance, tremors, palpitations, shortness of breath, and diarrhea. Examination findings include fever, tachycardia, brisk peripheral reflexes, dyspnea, tremors, vision changes, and may or may not include a goiter. Graves' disease (GD) may have unique manifestations including ophthalmopathy (exophthalmos), dermopathy (pretibial myxedema and generalized dermal thickening), and osteopathy (subperiosteal bone synthesis, swelling). Older patients may present with apathetic hyperthyroidism: a constellation of depression, weight loss, and slow atrial fibrillation. Untreated thyrotoxicosis can manifest with cardiac complications such as congestive heart failure (CHF), as well as arrhythmias, including atrial fibrillation. Other complications include osteoporosis, thyroid storm, and adverse pregnancy outcomes. The GD-specific manifestations can progress independent of the thyroid's disease course and may persist, despite obtaining the euthyroid state.[14]

Evaluation of Hyperthyroidism

The initial evaluation of hyperthyroidism includes a TSH as well as free T4. Total T3 is used to help diagnose conditions including estrogen excess and nonthyroidal illness but most laboratories only perform reflex to free T4 if the TSH is abnormal (**Fig. 1**).[15,16] Total T3 can also be helpful when elevated in the setting of normal free T4 with a low or undetectable TSH in mild hyperthyroidism.[17,18] Most cases of overt hyperthyroidism are primary hyperthyroidism that manifests as a suppressed or undetectable TSH in combination with an elevated free T4 level. Elevation of TSH, free T4, and total T3 is a rare instance and points to a cause of secondary hyperthyroidism such as TSH-producing pituitary adenomas or a thyroid hormone–resistant pituitary.[15,16] There can be interference with bloodwork accuracy aware and providers should be aware that biotin consumption (5–30 mg) can spuriously produce a pattern concerning for GD (low TSH, high T4, high thyroid-stimulating immunoglobulin [TSI]). Patients should not take biotin less than 48 hours prior to testing.[14]

GD has unique manifestations including exophthalmos, a large thyroid, and significant symptoms of hyperthyroidism. If all the aforementioned manifestations are present, further evaluation is unnecessary and the diagnosis of GD is conclusive. If there is concern for GD but the clinical symptoms are inconclusive, the evaluation should also include serum levels of TSI, which is 96% sensitive and 99% specific for GD. If etiology remains unclear after a negative TSI but suspicion for GD is still present, RAI uptake scan may be performed to further clarify etiology.[18] Increased uptake can be noted diffusely on the RAI uptake test in GD. Meanwhile, in toxic adenomas, the iodine uptake is focal on the uptake testing and in multinodular goiter, patchy areas of iodine uptake are typical. When the RAI uptake scan shows an absence of increased uptake, this indicates other causes of toxicosis such as medication induced and thyroiditis.

Secondary hyperthyroidism is rare and etiologies stem from either TSH-producing pituitary adenomas or a thyroid hormone–resistant pituitary. Both result in the unique laboratory finding of an elevated TSH in the presence of elevated free T4 and T3.[14,15] Further diagnosis can be confirmed by obtaining an MRI evaluating for a pituitary lesion.[18]

Treatment of Hyperthyroidism

Goals of treatment of hyperthyroidism include symptomatic control, as well as returning to and maintaining a euthyroid state. Achieving a euthyroid state, defined as a normal TSH assay, can be attempted with antithyroid drugs (ATDs), RAI therapy, or thyroidectomy. The symptoms of thyrotoxicosis (tachycardia, shortness of breath, hypertension, and so forth) can be controlled utilizing both specific and nonspecific beta-blockade in the form of atenolol and propranolol, respectively. ATD medications include methimazole (MMI) and propylthiouracil (PTU) and are preferred for pregnant patients and those with a high likelihood of remission,

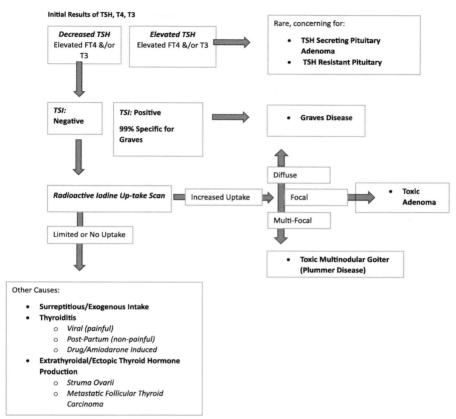

Fig. 1. Evaluation of hyperthyroidism/thyrotoxicosis in a nonpregnant patient.[14–18]

increased surgical risk, or a limited life expectancy. MMI is preferred over PTU, and optimal duration of ATD therapy involves a titration regimen over 12 to 18 months once remission is achieved. PTU is preferred for pregnant patients. Contraindications for ATDs include previous major adverse reactions, hepatic impairment, and present agranulocytosis.

RAI therapy is the preferred definitive treatment for most patients with hyperthyroidism. It is administered orally and selectively destroys overactive thyroid cells to normalize thyroid function but may result in hypothyroidism. RAI therapy is indicated for women planning a future pregnancy, patients with increased risk to surgery, those who have contraindications to ATDs, or are nonresponsive to ATDs. Lastly, thyroidectomy (total or subtotal) is indicated for women who are planning a future pregnancy, patients with large goiters or nodules, low uptake of RAI, and suspected or present thyroid malignancy.[19,20]

SUBCLINICAL THYROID DISEASE
Introduction

Subclinical thyroid disease is defined by the presence of abnormal TSH which is outside the normal range but with normal T4 and T3 levels. Subclinical thyroid disease is one of the most frequently encountered thyroid abnormalities with estimated prevalence of 3% to 12% for subclinical hypothyroidism (SCH) and 1% to 6% for subclinical hyperthyroidism (SCHr). It includes 2 entities: SCHr and SCH.[21] In SCHr, serum TSH concentrations are low or suppressed but free T4 and T3 concentrations are in the normal range, although a T3 is not needed for the diagnosis. In SCH, serum TSH concentrations are above the reference range of normal and free thyroid hormones are in the normal range.[22]

Diagnosis

Subclinical hyperthyroidism

SCHr is usually diagnosed when serum TSH is low or suppressed with normal thyroid hormone levels. However, not every person with a low serum TSH has SCHr.[22] Some healthy elderly people might have an age-related change in the TSH set point at the level of the hypothalamic-pituitary-axis resulting in a low serum TSH.[22–24] African American people tend to run a low TSH, which could be normal for them. According to the National Health and Nutrition Examination Survey (NHANES), 4% of African American people had serum TSH of less than 0.4 compared to 1.4% of Caucasians.[22,25] In some cases, low serum TSH concentrations are first seen in the first trimester of pregnancy related to thyroid stimulation by placental hCG, which has structural homology with TSH.[26] Low TSH can also be because of medical treatments such as high dose of glucocorticoids, dopamine, and amiodarone. Low serum TSH concentrations are more prevalent in cigarette smokers.[22] A low serum TSH value can also be transitory in younger patients and is often related to thyroiditis or mild GD, and it can be from toxic multinodular goiter and solitary autonomous nodules in elderly patients.[27]

Subclinical hypothyroidism

For the diagnosis of SCH, you will find a high TSH level with a normal free T4. SCH is classified as mild if TSH is 4.5 to 9 mIU/L and severe if the TSH is $\geq$10mIU/L.[22,28] Seventy-five percent of the patients with SCH have mild thyroid disease. The most common cause (60%–80% of cases) is from Hashimoto's thyroiditis.[22,29] Other physiologic/transient increases in serum TSH could be seen as part of nonthyroidal illness, subacute or postpartum thyroiditis, abnormal TSH isoforms, assay variability, or hydrophilic antibodies.[22,28,29] Other common causes are old age, obesity, impaired renal function, untreated adrenal insufficiency, and, in rare cases, isolated pituitary resistance to the thyroid hormone or TSH secreting adenomas.[22,29]

As mentioned earlier, there has been considerable debate regarding the reference range for serum TSH with age, gender, and ethnicity. TSH does not follow normal distribution and has diurnal variation.[27] According to NHANES III, a reference population had a narrower TSH range of 0.39 to 4.5mIU/L.[27] Higher TSH values have been demonstrated in the elderly, such that 14% of healthy individuals older than 80 years may have TSH values greater than 4.5, which could be normal for them.[22–24,27] These findings suggest some experts recommend age-specific TSH reference ranges.

Treatment

Treatment decisions are based predominantly on expert opinion due to lack of evidence of high-quality data (**Figs. 2** and **3**). In the setting of SCH, after diagnosis has been established with an elevated TSH and normal free T4, treatment can be further delineated with TSH levels (see **Fig. 2**). Similarly, after a diagnosis of SCHr has been established, treatment can be established using TSH levels and age using an individualized approach.

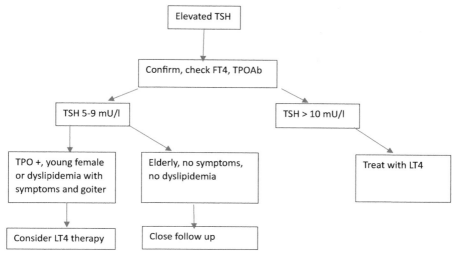

Fig. 2. Subclinical hypothyroidism treatment algorithm.[22,29]

Complications of Subclinical Thyroid Disease

Subclinical hyperthyroidism

SCHr is associated with almost double the risk of atrial fibrillation, and ischemic heart disease but not stroke, CHF, or cardiovascular (CV) mortality, and increased risk of fractures including hip fracture.[21,30–32]

Subclinical hypothyroidism

SCH may be associated with CV disease (heart failure, coronary artery disease events, and CV mortality) and may have cognitive impairment, nonspecific symptoms such as fatigue, and altered mood.[29,33–35]

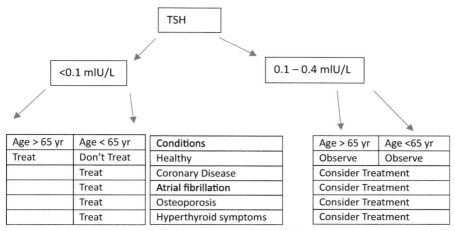

Fig. 3. Subclinical hyperthyroidism treatment algorithm.[22,29]

Conclusions

Subclinical thyroid disease is a common clinical problem routinely encountered during screening blood tests in asymptomatic patients. There are sufficient data to consider treatment for patients with SCHr who have a TSH less than 0.1 and people with SCH when TSH greater than 10. For most patients with TSH slightly above the normal range or mildly low TSH, an individualized approach to treatment and monitoring should be adopted based on patient's age, race, bodyweight, CV risk, and other comorbidities.

SICK EUTHYROID DISORDER

Introduction

Sick euthyroid disorders, also known as euthyroid sick syndrome (ESS), are most commonly seen in critical illness and are related to abnormal thyroid testing that is done in a hospital setting. It is related to nonthyroidal illnesses. ESS is a state of dysregulation where T3 and T4 are abnormal but there does not appear to be any abnormalities of the thyroid gland. It is not a true illness and is often seen in patients with critical illness, severe caloric deficits, severe sepsis, trauma, and after major surgeries.[36-38]

Diagnoses

Assessment of thyroid function in seriously ill patients is generally discouraged, unless there is a suspicion for thyroid dysfunction.[37-39] Laboratory analyses to obtain for ESS initially include serum TSH and free T4. Due to diminished hypothalamic function in patients who are seriously ill, TSH is expected to be low but detectable. If TSH levels are undetectable (<0.01) consider workup for thyrotoxicosis. There are different classifications of ESS including low T3 syndrome, low T4 syndrome, low T3 and T4 syndrome, high T4 syndrome, and others. Low T3 syndrome is the most common abnormality and is correlated with increased hospital length of stay. Low T3 and T4 syndrome is usually seen in patients in the intensive care unit.

A low serum T4 correlates with a bad prognosis and is associated with high mortality rates. Mortality rates of approximately 80% are seen with T4 levels less than 2 mcg/dL. High T4 syndrome can also be seen in patients receiving medications such as amiodarone or patients with liver diseases such as chronic hepatitis. It can precipitate hyperthyroidism in patients.

Management

Thyroid replacement is generally not indicated, but the underlying cause should be treated. If TSH is low and there is no suspicion for thyroid disease, TSH and free T4 can be re-evaluated after recovery from illness. If TSH is high but below 10, and the patient is recovering from their illness, a repeat TSH in 1 to 2 weeks is recommended.

Treatment could be considered in the following situations:

If TSH levels are between 10 and 20 and the patient has a low T4, cautious initiation of levothyroxine 12.5mcg/day could be done.

If TSH is above 20 and free T4 level is low, it is reasonable to start cautious repletion with half (0.8mcg/kg/day) the full levothyroxine replacement dose (1.6 mcg/kg/day).[40]

CLINICS CARE POINTS

- Euthyroid state is defined as a normal TSH between 0.45 and 4.12 based on the NHANES III reference.

- Hypothyroidism is defined as a high TSH and low free T4 and the goal of treatment is to have normal TSH assay with the use of levothyroxine.
- Hyperthyroidism is defined as a low TSH and high free T4. Treatment to achieve a goal euthyroid state is typically with ATDs, RAI therapy, or surgery.
- SCHr is defined as a low or suppressed TSH with a normal free T4.
- SCH is defined as a high TSH with a normal free T4.
- Sick euthyroid disorders are commonly seen in critical illness and are related to nonthyroidal illness.

DISCLOSURE

The authors have nothing to disclose.

REFERENCES

1. Wang D, Yu S, Ma C, et al. Reference intervals for thyroid-stimulating hormone, free thyroxine, and free triiodothyronine in elderly Chinese persons. Clin Chem Lab Med 2019;57(7):1044–52.
2. Andersson M, de Benoist B, Delange F, et al. Prevention and control of iodine deficiency in pregnant and lactating women and in children less than 2-years-old: conclusions and recommendations of the Technical Consultation. Publ Health Nutr 2007;10(12A):1606–11.
3. Chaker L, Bianco AC, Jonklaas J, et al. Hypothyroidism. Lancet 2017;390(10101):1550–62.
4. Baskin HJ, Cobin RH, Duick DS, et al. American Association of Clinical Endocrinologists medical guidelines for clinical practice for the evaluation and treatment of hyperthyroidism and hypothyroidism. Endocr Pract 2002;8:457–69.
5. Recommendation: Thyroid Dysfunction: Screening | United States Preventive Services Taskforce. 2015. Available at: www.uspreventiveservicestaskforce.org;. [Accessed 1 May 2024] https://www.uspreventiveservicestaskforce.org/uspstf/recommendation/thyroid-dysfunction-screening.
6. Garber JR, Cobin RH, Gharib H, et al. Clinical practice guidelines for hypothyroidism in adults: cosponsored by the American Association of Clinical Endocrinologists and the American Thyroid Association [published correction appears in Endocr Pract. 2013 Jan-Feb;19(1):175]. Endocr Pract 2012;18(6):988–1028.
7. Ban Y, Greenberg DA, Davies TF, et al. Linkage analysis of thyroid antibody production: evidence for shared susceptibility to clinical autoimmune thyroid disease. J Clin Endocrinol Metab 2008;93(9):3589–96.
8. Kim MI. Hypothyroidism in Older Adults. In: Feingold KR, Anawalt B, Blackman MR, et al, editors. Endotext [Internet]. South Dartmouth (MA): MDText.com, Inc.; 2020. p. 2000. Available at: https://www.ncbi.nlm.nih.gov/books/NBK279005/.
9. Sforza N, Rosenfarb J, Rujelman R, et al. Hypothyroidism in hospitalized elderly patients: a sign of worse prognosis. J Endocrinol Invest 2017;40(12):1303–10.
10. Jonklaas J, Bianco AC, Bauer AJ, et al. Guidelines for the treatment of hypothyroidism: prepared by the american thyroid association task force on thyroid hormone replacement. Thyroid 2014;24(12):1670–751.
11. Roos A, Linn-Rasker SP, van Domburg RT, et al. The starting dose of levothyroxine in primary hypothyroidism treatment: a prospective, randomized, double-blind trial

[published correction appears in Arch Intern Med. 2005 Oct 24;165(19):2227]. Arch Intern Med 2005;165(15):1714–20.

12. Koulouri O, Moran C, Halsall D, et al. Pitfalls in the measurement and interpretation of thyroid function tests. Best Pract Res Clin Endocrinol Metab 2013;27(6): 745–62.

13. Wood MD, Delate T, Clark M, et al. An evaluation of the potential drug interaction between warfarin and levothyroxine. J Thromb Haemost 2014. https://doi.org/10.1111/jth.12626.

14.. Lee GA, Masharani U. Disorders of the thyroid gland. In: Lalwani AK, editor. Current diagnosis & treatment Otolaryngology - Head & neck surgery. 4th edition. New York, NY: McGraw-Hill Education; 2020. p. 685–706.

15. Kravets I. Hyperthyroidism: Diagnosis and Treatment. Am Fam Physician 2016; 93(5):363–70.

16. Davey RX, Clarke MI, Webster AR. Thyroid function testing based on assay of thyroid-stimulating hormone: assessing an algorithm's reliability. Med J Aust 1996;164(6):329–32.

17.. Bakerman S, Bakerman P, Strausbauch P. Bakerman's ABC's of interpretive laboratory data. 5th edition. Phoenix, AZ: Interpretive Laboratory Data, Inc.; 2014.

18. Ross DS, Burch HB, Cooper DS, et al. 2016 American Thyroid Association Guidelines for Diagnosis and Management of Hyperthyroidism and Other Causes of Thyrotoxicosis. Thyroid 2016;26(10):1343–421 [published correction appears in Thyroid. 2017 Nov;27(11):1462].

19. Abraham P, Avenell A, McGeoch SC, et al. Antithyroid drug regimen for treating Graves' hyperthyroidism. Cochrane Database Syst Rev 2010;(1):CD003420. Accessed 18 December 2023.

20. Bahn Chair RS, Burch HB, Cooper DS, et al. Hyperthyroidism and other causes of thyrotoxicosis: management guidelines of the American Thyroid Association and American Association of Clinical Endocrinologists. Thyroid 2011;21(6):593–646 [published correction appears in Thyroid. 2011;21(10):1169] [published correction appears in Thyroid. 2012 Nov;22(11):1195].

21. Ettleson MD. Cardiovascular outcomes in subclinical thyroid disease: an update. Curr Opin Endocrinol Diabetes Obes 2023;30(5):218–24.

22. Cooper DS, Biondi B. Subclinical thyroid disease. Lancet 2012;379:1142–54.

23. Bremner AP, Feddema P, Leedman PJ, et al. Age-related changes in thyroid function: a longitudinal study of a community-based cohort. J Clin Endocrinol Metab 2012;97(5):1554–62.

24. Surks MI, Hollowell JG. Age-specific distribution of serum thyrotropin and antithyroidantibodies in the US population: implications for the prevalence of subclinical hypothyroidism. J Clin Endocrinol Metab 2007;92(12):4575–82.

25. Hollowell JG, Staehling NW, Flanders WD, et al. Serum TSH, T4,and thyroid antibodies in the United States population (1988 to1994): National Health and Nutrition Examination Survey (NHANES III). J Clin Endocrinol Metab 2002;87:489–99.

26. Glinoer D, De Nayer P, Robyn C, et al. Serum levels of intact human chorionic gonadotropin (HCG) andits free alpha and beta subunits, in relation to maternal thyroid stimulation during normal pregnancy. J Endocrinol Invest 1993;16:881–8.

27. Abraham-Nordling M, Torring O, Lantz M, et al. Incidence of hyperthyroidism in Stockholm, Sweden, 2003–2005. Eur J Endocrinol 2008;158:823–7.

28. Peeters RP. Subclinical hypothyroidism. N Engl J Med 2017;376(26):2556–65.

29. Biondi B, Cappola AR, Cooper DS. Subclinical Hypothyroidism: A Review. JAMA 2019;322(2):153–60.

30. Baumgartner C, da Costa BR, Collet TH, et al. Thyroid function within the normal range, subclinical hypothyroidism, and the risk of atrial fibrillation. Circulation 2017;136:2100–16.
31. Sohn SY, Lee E, Lee MK, et al. The association of overt and subclinical hyperthyroidism with the risk of cardiovascular events and cardiovascular mortality: meta-analysis and systematic review of cohort studies. Endocrinol Metab (Seoul) 2020; 35:786–800.
32. Blum MR, Bauer DC, Collet TH, et al. Subclinical thyroid dysfunction and fracture risk: a meta-analysis. JAMA 2015;313(20):2055–65.
33. Huang M, Yang S, Ge G, et al. Effects of thyroid dysfunction and the thyroid stimulating hormone levels on the risk of atrial fibrillation: a systematic review and dose-response meta-analysis from cohort studies. Endocr Pract 2022;28:822–31.
34. Chaker L, Baumgartner C, den Elzen WP, et al. Subclinical hypothyroidis and the risk of stroke events and fatal stroke: an individual participant data analysis. J Clin Endocrinol Metab 2015;100:2181–91.
35. Moon S, Kim MJ, Yu JM, et al. Subclinical hypothyroidism and the risk of Cardiovascular disease and all-cause mortality: a meta-analysis of prospective cohort studies. Thyroid 2018;28:1101–10.
36. Gutch M, Kumar S, Gupta KK. Prognostic Value of Thyroid Profile in Critical Care Condition. Indian J Endocrinol Metab 2018;22(3):387–91.
37. Vitiello R, Perisano C, Covino M, et al. Euthyroid sick syndrome in hip fractures: Valuation of vitamin D and parathyroid hormone axis. Injury 2020;51(Suppl 3): S13–6.
38. Docter R, Krenning EP, de Jong M, et al. The sick euthyroid syndrome: changes in thyroid hormone serum parameters and hormone metabolism. Clin Endocrino 1993;39:499–518.
39. Wang YF, Heng JF, Yan J, et al. Relationship between disease severity and thyroid function in Chinese patients with euthyroid sick syndrome. Medicine (Baltim) 2018;97(31):e11756.
40. Smallridge RC. Metabolic and anatomic thyroid emergencies: a review. Crit Care Med 1992;20(2):276–91.

Adrenal Pathologies

Katherine Johnson, MD

KEYWORDS

- Adrenal mass • Cortisol • Aldosterone • Adrenal insufficiency • Pheochromocytoma

KEY POINTS

- Adrenal nodules/masses are commonly found incidentally on imaging and require assessment of cancer risk and autonomous hormonal secretion.
- Clinicians should consider assessment for pheochromocytoma, hyperaldosteronism, and hypercortisolism in all adrenal masses, and they should additionally consider evaluating for congenital adrenal hyperplasia in cases of bilateral adrenal hyperplasia.
- Adrenal crisis is a condition of inadequate cortisol production and is a life-threatening condition that should be treated immediately with intravenous steroids and fluids.

INTRODUCTION

The adrenal glands produce several hormones necessary for regulation of metabolism, blood pressure, stress response, and sexual development. To understand adrenal dysfunction, it is important to have a basic understanding of normal adrenal function. The adrenal gland is divided into 2 zones, the cortex and the medulla. Each zone secretes different hormones that perform specific functions within the body. The key hormones produced by the adrenal cortex include cortisol, aldosterone, dehydroepiandrosterone, and androgenic steroids. The main hormones secreted by the adrenal medulla include epinephrine and norepinephrine.

Primary care providers should be able to recognize and perform an initial evaluation for adrenal pathologies that include adrenal insufficiency, pheochromocytoma, Cushing's syndrome, and Conn syndrome. The presence of unilateral or bilateral adrenal mass or hyperplasia is a common cause of hypersecretion of adrenal hormones, but these masses may also be non-secretory. Incidental adrenal masses (incidentalomas) are common findings and primary care clinicians should be aware of basic adrenal incidentaloma evaluation as well as imaging findings concerning for malignancy.

PHEOCHROMOCYTOMA
Introduction

Pheochromocytoma is a rare tumor that results in excess production of epinephrine and/or norepinephrine catecholamines by the adrenal medulla or, less often, a

Diplomate of ABOM, Diplomate of ABCL, Department of Family Medicine, Self Regional Healthcare, 155 Academy Avenue, Greenwood, SC 29646, USA
E-mail address: Katherine.Johnson@selfregional.org

Prim Care Clin Office Pract 51 (2024) 417–430
https://doi.org/10.1016/j.pop.2024.03.005
0095-4543/24/© 2024 Elsevier Inc. All rights reserved.
primarycare.theclinics.com

paraganglion. The catecholamine production is commonly in cyclical bursts. Up to 14% of adrenal masses found incidentally on imaging studies are pheochromocytomas.[1]

Symptoms

Pheochromocytomas may cause persistent or paroxysmal hypertension that can be difficult to control with blood pressure medications. Other symptoms include severe headaches, palpitations, diaphoresis, tremors, and anxiety.[2]

Evaluation

All pheochromocytomas have Hounsfield Units (HU) >10, so adrenal masses with HU </=10 do not need further assessment for pheochromocytoma.[1] Initial screening test for pheochromocytoma is plasma metanephrines or 24-hour urine collection for fractionate metanephrines and catecholamines.[2] Results of 2 to 4 × upper limit of the normal reference range is considered abnormal. They are localized by computed tomography (CT) or MRI of the adrenal glands and abdomen. In some cases, PET scan may also be useful.[2]

Treatment

Once a pheochromocytoma is identified, patients should be referred to endocrinology and surgery for further management. Laparoscopic and adrenal-sparing surgical intervention following preoperative alpha-blockade is the treatment of choice and usually curative.[2] In malignant pheochromocytomas, radiotherapy and chemotherapy are palliative treatment options.[2]

HYPERALDOSTERONISM
Introduction

Aldosterone is a mineralocorticoid hormone that plays a central role in regulating blood pressure, pH, and electrolytes (sodium and potassium). Primary hyperaldosteronism is due to dysfunction of the adrenal gland. Primary hyperaldosteronism is the most common form of secondary hypertension (HTN), with an estimated prevalence of 4% of hypertensive patients in primary care.[3] Aldosterone-producing adrenal adenomas account for around 40% and idiopathic hyperaldosteronism for around 60% of primary hyperaldosteronism cases.[3] When the cause of hyperaldosteronism is an adrenal tumor/adenoma, the disease is called Conn syndrome.

Symptoms

Hyperaldosteronism causes sodium retention, plasma renin suppression, HTN, increased CV risk, and increased potassium excretion, leading to variable degrees of hypokalemia that may present as myalgias, muscle spasms, or weakness.[3]

Evaluation

Initial screening should be done with a morning (8 AM) aldosterone and plasma renin activity level.[3] An aldosterone to plasma renin activity ratio of 20:1 suggests excessive aldosterone secretion. Positive findings (elevated aldosterone and low renin) warrant computed tomography (CT) adrenal/abdominal as initial imaging and further evaluation by an endocrine specialist.

Treatment

Medical management versus surgical management should be considered. In the setting of unilateral adrenal nodules, laparoscopic surgical resection is preferred. If the surgery is deemed inappropriate/undesired or if there is bilateral adrenal disease, medical management with mineralocorticoid receptor antagonists is preferred. Spironolactone is considered first-line therapy, but eplerenone may be considered if spironolactone side effects preclude its use.[4]

HYPERCORTISOLISM
Introduction

Cortisol is a glucocorticoid hormone produced by the adrenal gland and helps regulate blood pressure, metabolic functions, blood glucose, immune function, and the sleep/wake cycle. It is released during times of stress. It is produced in the zona fasciculata of the adrenal gland under regulation from the hypothalamic pituitary adrenal (HPA) axis. Cortisol-releasing hormone (CRH) produced within the hypothalamus triggers adrenocorticotropic hormone (ACTH) release from the anterior pituitary gland. ACTH in turn drives the production of cortisol within the adrenal gland. The hypothalamus and the pituitary gland regulate cortisol levels through a negative feedback loop. If there is an excess or paucity of cortisol, the hypothalamus and pituitary change the amount of CRH and ACTH released, respectively.

Cushing's syndrome (CS) is defined as a state of elevated plasma cortisol levels that leads to classic syndrome that may include skin fragility, easy bruising, purple striae, muscle loss and myopathy, weakness, immunosuppression, osteopenia, and fat deposition on face, abdomen, and cervical pad.[5] The most common cause is from intake of exogenous steroid such as prednisone or dexamethasone.[5] When CS is due to excessive ACTH production in the pituitary gland, it is referred to as Cushing's disease (CD), and is the most common cause of endogenous CS, accounting for 65% of cases.[5] Other less common endogenous causes of CS include adrenal tumors and adrenal hyperplasia, aka primary hypercortisolism (30% of endogenous CS).[5] ACTH-secreting tumors of malignant or neuroendocrine origin (ie, small cell lung cancer) make up the smallest percentage of endogenous CS cases at 5%.[5]

Classic CS features may not be easily appreciated or present at all with adrenal tumors as more subtle hypercortisolism is often associated with a hormonally active adrenal nodule. Hypercortisolism without the clinical/phenotypical features of CS has varied names including "subclinical Cushing's Syndrome," "subclinical hypercortisolism (SH)," "possible/mild autonomous cortisol secretion (pACS/MACS)." For the remaining discussion, the term "mild autonomous cortisol secretion (MACS)" will be utilized. Approximately 10% (range 1%–29%) of patients with adrenal incidentaloma will have serologic findings of MACS.[1] Patients with MACS can present with comorbidities associated with cortisol excess including cardiovascular disease, hypertension, insulin resistance, dyslipidemia, obesity, oligomenorrhea, fatty liver disease, and osteoporosis.[6,7]

Evaluation and Diagnosis

There is no single preferred diagnostic test when there is clinical suspicion for CS. Before undergoing laboratory evaluation, a careful history should exclude exogenous glucocorticoid intake. Initial screening tests include the Late Night Salivary Cortisol Test, 24-hour urinary free cortisol test, and dexamethasone suppression test (DST) (**Box 1**).[8]

It is important to note that electronic health record (EHR)lab results may not have set normal parameters for a cortisol level that is post dexamethasone dosing. Therefore, the clinician must know to interpret the cortisol DST result considering the dexamethasone level and not rely on the normal range for cortisol noted on the lab results. Interpretation of initial results and further evaluation is best done in consultation with an endocrinologist.

> **Box 1**
> **Instructions for 1-mg dexamethasone suppression test**
>
> Step 1: On night prior to blood draw: Take 1 mg dexamethasone between 11:00 PM and Midnight.
>
> Step 2: Subsequent morning: obtain cortisol level between 8 and 9 AM[a]
>
> [a]Consider co-testing of dexamethasone level to ensure veracity of test.

Once biochemical evidence of hypercortisolism is found on the initial screening tests, early morning ACTH levels should be measured. The ACTH can help guide where to image, with normal to high levels of ACTH suggesting a pituitary cause and a pituitary MRI should be performed.[8] Low ACTH levels (<10 pg/mL) suggest an adrenal cause of CS and an adrenal CT or MRI should be obtained.

Treatment

Treatment should involve multiple specialists including endocrinology, oncology, and surgery and include surgical tumor resection, medications, and radiation therapy. Medical therapies such as osilodrostat, metyrapone, and ketoconazole can be used to block steroidogenesis in the adrenal gland. These therapies can rapidly normalize serum cortisol levels. Mifepristone is a potent glucocorticoid receptor blocker and FDA approved for treatment of hyperglycemia in the setting of hypercortisolism. For CD with an inoperable tumor, pasireotide and cabergoline function to block ACTH centrally and shrink the pituitary adenoma, but are less effective at normalizing cortisol levels. Bilateral adrenalectomy may be recommended to stabilize patients with CS that is severe and/or resistant to treatment because it can rapidly relieve hypercortisolism.[5]

Prognosis/Surveillance

Patients with CS require lifelong monitoring that includes biochemical testing. Primary care doctors should monitor these patients closely in consultation with endocrinology.

CLINICS CARE POINTS

- If pheochromocytoma is considered, initial screening is plasma metanephrine levels.
- Initial screening for an aldosterone-secreting tumor is a morning renin and aldosterone level.
- Cushing's syndrome is a nonspecific condition of cortisol excess with the most common cause being use of exogenous steroids.
- Treatments of CS include surgical and medical therapies depending on the underlying cause.

ADRENAL ADENOMAS
Adrenal Masses, Unilateral

Approximately 4% of abdominal imaging reveals an adrenal nodule/mass, and frequency increases with advancing age. True prevalence is not known, but postmortem studies estimate this to be around 6%.[1,9] Adrenal nodules are often found incidentally on imaging, and thus are commonly referred to as "incidentalomas." Adrenal nodules found during cancer surveillance are not technically incidental findings, and in these cases, evaluation of metastatic disease is paramount. All incidental masses require assessment for both cancer risk and inappropriate hormonal activity. Reported prevalence of specific conditions diagnosed during evaluation varies widely due to differing selection criteria and different definitions of hormone excess. See **Table 1** for estimated breakdown.[10]

Oncologic Assessment

Adrenal incidentaloma is defined as an adrenal lesion detected on imaging originally performed for some other indication than assessment for adrenal disease. Typically, these lesions are >1 cm in size. Over 90% of adrenal incidentalomas are benign.[2] All adrenal masses require dedicated adrenal imaging, ideally non-contrasted abdominal CT if not already completed. Homogenous lesions with Hounsfield Units (HU) </=10 are considered very lipid-rich and indicate very low likelihood of malignancy. These masses require no further imaging studies.[9,10]

Masses found to be >10 HU on unenhanced CT require more in-depth analysis and risk stratification. Statistically, these lesions are still likely benign. Further imaging with MRI or CT imaging with contrast washout protocol may be considered.[9] However, to date, there is not high-quality evidence to support the most effective imaging choice after unenhanced CT imaging. The 2023 European guidelines on adrenal nodules suggest that ideally, referral to a multidisciplinary team for continued assessment is recommended. Adrenal carcinoma is rare, and typically only non-homogenous lesions of >4 cm or lesions of >4 cm with HU of greater than 10 are considered high risk enough for surgical excision. See **Fig. 1** for recommended flow chart, as published by the 2023 European workgroup on adrenal incidentalomas.

Fine needle biopsy is not recommended for diagnosis of primary adrenal carcinoma, but this may be utilized in a patient with known primary malignancy elsewhere if a new adrenal mass is identified and radiographic appearance is consistent with metastatic disease.[1] Characteristics of metastatic adrenal disease are listed in **Box 2**.

A biopsy may also be considered if infection is suspected, particularly if an infiltrative organism such as mycobacterium or fungal organism is suspected. Characteristics that increase risk of infiltrate infection would be an immunocompromised status or

Table 1
Etiology of adrenal tumors identified initially as adrenal incidentaloma[10]

Hormonal:	
• Nonfunctioning	• 40%–70%
• Mild autonomous cortisol secretion (MACS)	• 20%–50%
• Primary aldosteronism	• 2%–5%
• Overt Cushing's syndrome	• 1%–4%
• Pheochromocytoma	• 1%–5%
Oncologic	
• Adrenocortical carcinoma	• 0.4%-4%
• Other malignant mass (mostly metastasis)	• 3%–7%
Benign	
• Myelolipoma	• 3%–6%
• Cysts/Pseudocyst	• 1%
• Ganglioneuroma	• 1%
• Schwannoma	• <1%
• Hemorrhage	• <1%

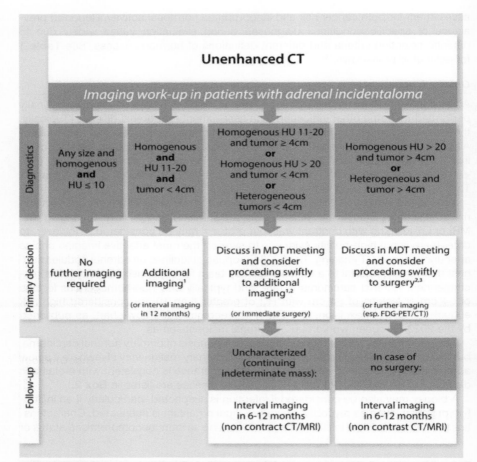

Fig. 1. Unenhanced computed tomography. *Eur J Endocrinol*, volume 189, Issue 1, July 2023, Pages G1–G42, https://doi.org/10.1093/ejendo/lvad066.

patients having lived or traveled to endemic areas. Prior to any biopsy, pheochromocytoma should be ruled out.

If imaging characteristics suggest primary adrenal carcinoma, a cancer-focused surgery should be obtained rather than biopsy, but this ought to be directed by the

---

Box 2
Radiographic characteristics of metastatic adrenal disease[1,9,10]

10 HU

Bilateral adrenal involvement

Heterogenous appearance (irregular borders and lack of smooth contours

>/=4 cm

Low absolute washout percentage

---

expertise of an endocrine surgeon since biopsy may be considered if the mass is deemed unresectable.[9]

Other benign pathologies of adrenal cysts, adrenal hemorrhage, and myelolipoma are easily identified on imaging and do not require further evaluation.

BILATERAL ADRENAL MASSES OR BILATERAL ADRENAL HYPERPLASIA

When multiple adrenal lesions are noted on imaging, the same assessment framework should be used as for unilateral lesions.[10] Malignancy risk for each individual lesion should be assessed, and assessment for hormonal activity should be identical to that of a unilateral lesion.

Evaluation for hormonal excess should include consideration for cortisol, catecholamine, and aldosterone excess, and evaluation is identical to that of a unilateral adenoma. However, for bilateral adenomas and hyperplasia, additional testing of 17-hydroxyprogesterone is indicated to exclude congenital adrenal hyperplasia (CAH) due to 21-hydroxylase deficiency.[9]

HORMONAL EVALUATION

Three conditions should be considered in all patients with an adrenal mass: pheochromocytoma, primary hyperaldosteronism, and hypercortisolism. Each of these conditions is discussed separately in this article (*see preceding sections*).

CLINICS CARE POINTS

- Adrenal incidentalomas should be evaluated for oncologic risk, ideally with unenhanced CT scan.
- Unenhanced CT scan with results a homogenous mass of ≤ 10 Hounsfield Units is almost certainly non-malignant.
- Adrenal masses found during cancer surveillance are not truly incidentalomas, and adrenal metastasis should be thoroughly ruled out.
- Familiarity of characteristics associated with malignancy is necessary for clinicians, as this may affect choice of conservative management, referral, or urgent consideration of biopsy.
- All adrenal nodules require hormonal evaluation for consideration of aldosterone and cortisol secretion and to rule out pheochromocytoma
- Adrenal nodules with HU <10 do NOT need to be evaluated for pheochromocytoma

---

ADRENAL INSUFFICIENCY
Introduction

Adrenal insufficiency is a rare disorder. Adrenocorticotropic hormone (ACTH), secreted by the anterior pituitary gland, stimulates synthesis of cortisol and androgens in the adrenal cortex. Therefore, the adrenal gland is dependent on an intact HPA axis for appropriate production and regulation of cortisol. Low adrenal hormone output due to ATCH deficiency is referred to as central adrenal insufficiency (CAI). ACTH deficiency with CAI may be isolated or occur in conjunction with other pituitary hormone deficiencies. Primary adrenal insufficiency (also known as Addison's disease) is due to a failure of the adrenal gland itself, despite adequate hormonal stimulation by ACTH levels. The most common cause of primary adrenal insufficiency is autoimmune disorders, but it can also be related to infections, tumors, or genetic factors.[11] Primary adrenal insufficiency (PAI) in children is most likely due to congenital adrenal hyperplasia (CAH), occurring in approximately 1 out of 14,000 live births.[12] Children who are born with CAH are missing an essential enzyme necessary to produce cortisol, aldosterone, or both. These children often also experience excess androgen production, which can lead to male characteristics in girls and precocious puberty in boys. In severe cases, infants with CAH may suffer from ambiguous genitalia, vomiting, dehydration, and failure to thrive.

Symptoms of Adrenal Insufficiency

Signs and symptoms of chronic adrenal insufficiency are often nonspecific and include weight loss, poor appetite, nausea and vomiting, diarrhea, fatigue, weakness, darkening of skin due to melanocyte stimulation (only in primary adrenal insufficiency), abdominal pain, weakness, fatigue, anorexia, dizziness, and orthostatic hypotension.[11]

Although adrenal insufficiency usually develops over time, it can also appear suddenly as an acute adrenal failure (adrenal crisis). Acute adrenal insufficiency has similar symptoms, but the consequences are more serious, including life-threatening shock, seizures, and coma. It is important to recognize acute adrenal insufficiency because treatment may be life-saving. Therefore, in discussing evaluation and treatment of adrenal insufficiency, the author will discuss chronic adrenal insufficiency and acute adrenal insufficiency separately.

Chronic Adrenal Insufficiency Evaluation

The evaluation and diagnosis of adrenal insufficiency can be challenging and it is important to properly differentiate between CAI and PAI. While not confirmatory, hyperkalemia is indicative of PAI, as the renin-angiotensin-aldosterone system is intact in CAI.[13] Initial evaluation of suspected adrenal insufficiency includes screening for current exogenous corticosteroid use, as it is the most common cause of adrenal insufficiency.[13] Once steroid-related adrenal insufficiency is ruled out, further testing should be performed. The cosyntropin stimulation test (AKA: ACTH stimulation test or Short Synacthen test) is considered the optimal diagnostic test. However, this test requires corticotropin be given via intravenous (IV) or intramuscular with cortisol levels being drawn at 30 or 60 min after corticotropin injection. This is not feasible for many primary care clinicians. Therefore, morning cortisol with concurrent or subsequent ACTH testing is a common initial screening test.[14] Cortisol levels should be checked between 8 and 9 AM with levels of less than 5 mcg/dL iconsistent with adrenal insufficiency and a cortisol level greater than 15 mcg essentially rules out AI. An elevated ACTH level with low cortisol indicates PAI, whereas a low or inappropriately normal ACTH value with low cortisol indicates CAI. When test results are equivocal, endocrine consultation is recommended (**Table 2**).[13]

If PAI is diagnosed or highly suspected, measurement of anti-21-Hydroxylase antibodies should be obtained for the diagnosis of autoimmune adrenalitis, the most common cause.[8] In patients with confirmed primary AI, measurement of plasma renin and aldosterone levels is necessary to determine concurrent mineralocorticoid deficiency.[9] If the diagnosis of CAI is made, a contrast-enhanced MRI of the sella turcica is useful

Table 2
Serologic differentiation of primary adrenal insufficiency and central adrenal insufficiency[13,14]

	Primary Adrenal Insufficiency	Central Adrenal Insufficiency
Cortisol	Low	Low
ACTH	High	Low/inappropriately normal

to detect pituitary masses and infectious or lymphocytic central nervous system disease.[13]

Abnormalities in corticosteroid-binding globulin (CBG) and albumin may affect the total cortisol levels. This is commonly found in patients on estrogen therapy (causing high CBG) or those with cirrhosis or nephrotic syndrome (low CBG). In these patients, free cortisol is an alternative. For women taking estrogen, 1 option is to discontinue the oral estrogen for 6 to 8 weeks and then perform the cosyntropin stimulation test.[14]

TREATMENT OF CHRONIC ADRENAL INSUFFICIENCY

All individuals with adrenal insufficiency require glucocorticoid replacement therapy.[13] Hydrocortisone is generally preferred, but other regimines can be utilized (**Table 3**).[12,14] Hormonal monitoring by serum testing is not recommended to drive therapy. Treatment should be initiated and adjusted to achieve clinical improvement under endocrinology supervision.

MINERALOCORTICOID REPLACEMENT IN CHRONIC PRIMARY ADRENAL INSUFFICIENCY

In patients with central CAI, unlike in PAI, mineralocorticoid (aldosterone) production is not impacted (**Table 4**).[12]

Fludrocortisone is the drug of choice for patients with confirmed aldosterone deficiency. Dosing should be .05 to 0.1 mg daily. Typically, if patient is using hydrocortisone or cortisone acetate, the starting dose is 0.05 mg since these agents have some small amount of mineralocorticoid activity. If the patient is taking prednisolone, the starting dose is typically fludrocortisone 0.1 mg daily.[14]

Mineralocorticoid replacement should be adjusted based on both clinical and biochemical markers. Clinically, orthostatic hypotension, salt craving, and postural dizziness should prompt consideration of increasing medication dose. Development of hypertension and edema typically indicate excessive mineralocorticoid replacement and fludrocortisone dose should be deescalated.[8,9] Biochemical markers for dose adjustment should include serum sodium, potassium, creatinine, and renin levels. Either plasma renin activity (PRA) or direct renin concentration (DRC) can be used for monitoring. The PRA aim should be in the upper limit of normal, and the DRC goal should be within normal range or slightly above.[15]

DEHYDROEPIANDROSTERONE REPLACEMENT IN CHRONIC PRIMARY ADRENAL INSUFFICIENCY

The Endocrine Society suggests consideration of DHEA supplementation (typically 25–50 mg/day) in patients with primary AI and low libido, depressed mood, and/or low energy levels. If the patient does not report a sustained improvement in their symptoms after 6 months, the treatment should be stopped.[12,14]

ACUTE ADRENAL INSUFFICIENCY (ALSO KNOWN AS ADRENAL CRISIS, ADDISONIAN CRISIS)
Introduction

Adrenal crisis occurs when the adrenal glands cannot respond appropriately to an acute stimulus requiring higher cortisol production. Clinically, patients present with refractory hypotension and volume depletion. Nonspecific findings of chronic adrenal insufficiency (anorexia, nausea, weakness, fatigue) and more severe lethargy, coma, and confusion are also often appreciated, particularly prior to shock. Acute Adrenal

Table 3
Glucocorticoid replacement dosing[12,14]

Drug	Total Daily Dose	Dosing Strategy	Notes
Hydrocortisone (fixed dosing)	15–25 mg	2 dose regimens: • 2/3 daily dose given in morning • 1/3 daily dose in afternoon, (approx. 2 h after lunch) 3 dose regimen: • Decreasing doses at morning, midday, and early evening	First dose should be highest dose and may be administered immediately upon waking
Hydrocortisone (weight-based dosing)	10–12 mg/m² body surface area	2 dose regimen: • 2/3 daily dose given in morning • 1/3 daily dose in afternoon (approx. 2 h after lunch) 3 dose regimen: • Decreasing doses at morning, midday, and early evening	First dose should be highest dose and may be administered immediately upon waking
Cortisone Acetate	20–35 mg	2 dose regimen: • 2/3 daily dose given in morning • 1/3 daily dose in afternoon (approx. 2 h after lunch) 3 dose regimen: • Decreasing doses at morning, midday, and early evening	First dose should be highest dose and may be administered immediately upon waking
Prednisolone	3–5 mg/d	1 dose regimen: • Take full dose upon waking 2 dose regimen • 70%–80% of daily dose in morning upon waking • Remainder at bedtime	This medication choice is reserved for patients having difficulty with multi day regimens and is not considered first line.

Table 4 Glucocorticoid and mineralocorticoid replacement dependent on type of adrenal insufficiency[12]		
	Primary Adrenal Insufficiency	**Central Adrenal Insufficiency**
Glucocorticoid necessary	Yes	Yes
Mineralocorticoid necessary	Yes	No

crisis is a life-threatening emergency that requires immediate treatment and should be suspected in patients who present with vasodilatory shock. Early recognition and correct management are mandatory to avoid significant morbidity and mortality. Treatment should never be delayed for diagnostic testing.

In 2019, Rushworth and colleagues set out the following definition for adrenal crisis: "An acute deterioration in health status associated with absolute hypotension (systolic blood pressure <100 mm Hg) or relative hypotension (systolic blood pressure >/ =20 mm Hg lower than usual), with features that resolve within 1 to 2 hours after parenteral glucocorticoid administration."[16]

In pediatric populations, hypotension may be harder to accurately identify during emergency situations. In this scenario, adrenal crisis was defined as "as an acute deterioration in health status associated with an acute hemodynamic disturbance (hypotension or sinus tachycardia relative to age-related normative data) or a marked electrolyte abnormality (eg, hyponatremia, hyperkalemia, or hypoglycemia) not attributable to another illness."[16]

Precipitating Factors for Acute Adrenal Insufficiency

Recent history is vital in identifying patients who may need aggressive glucocorticoid treatment prior to definitive diagnosis. Factors that should increase the clinicians concern include as follows:[16]

1. Known chronic adrenal insufficiency with sudden clinical worsening, recent major stressor (physical or psychological), or signs/symptoms of infection.
2. Recent changes in glucocorticoid and/or mineralocorticoid dosing.
3. Concern for acute adrenal gland destruction (hemorrhage or infarct), particularly in patients taking anticoagulants.
4. Head/pituitary injuries causing acute HPA axis disruption.
5. Change (addition or deletion) of non-adrenal-related medications.
   a. Immune checkpoint inhibitors
   b. Cytochrome P450 3A4 (CYP3A4) inducers (carbamazepine, phenytoin, St. John's wort, rifampicin, etc.)
   c. CYP3A4 inhibitors ("azole" medications, grapefruit juice, clarithromycin, ritonavir, etc.)
6. Undiagnosed coexisting thyrotoxicosis or use of thyroxine in hypoadrenalism.

Adrenal Crisis Treatment

Acute adrenal crisis is treated with IV glucocorticoid therapy (hydrocortisone is the preferred agent) and fluid resuscitation to correct hypovolemia and hyponatremia. Dextrose-containing fluids can be used to treat hypoglycemia. See **Table 5** for specific dosing recommendations.[16] If hypotension and hyponatremia is refractory to parenteral hydrocortisone and fluid administration, it suggests an alternative diagnosis to adrenal crisis.

Table 5
Adrenal crisis treatment in adults and pediatrics[16]

Drug	Initial Dose	Subsequent Doses	Notes
Hydrocortisone[a] (Adults) (Preferred agent)	100 mg intravenous (IV) or intramuscular (IM)	• 50 mg every 6 h	Provide 1 L normal saline in first h and subsequent crystalloid fluids according to resuscitative needs
Hydrocortisone[a] (Pediatric) (Preferred agent)	50 mg IV/IM per square meter of body-surface area	• 12.5–25 mg per square meter every 6 h	Provide 20 mL/kg of body weight bolus of normal saline in first h and subsequent crystalloid fluids according to resuscitative needs
Dexamethasone (Adults)	4 mg every 24 h	• Not applicable	Provide 1 L normal saline in first h and subsequent crystalloid fluids according to resuscitative needs
Methylprednisolone (Adults)	40 mg every 24 h	Not Applicable	Provide 1 L normal saline in first h and subsequent crystalloid fluids according to resuscitative needs
Prednisolone (Adults)	25 mg bolus	• 25 mg q 8 h for total dose of 75 mg in first 24 h • 50 mg every 24 h subsequently	Provide 1 L normal saline in first h and subsequent crystalloid fluids according to resuscitative needs

[a] If primary adrenal insufficiency (AI) is already established, fludrocortisone replacement is considered at time of initial hydrocortisone dose.

Once the patient has stabilized, the steroid can be tapered and converted to an oral maintenance regimen. The precipitating cause of adrenal crisis should be identified and treated appropriately. Treatment should be initiated immediately, when suspected, and prior to completion of the evaluation.

PREVENTION OF ACUTE ADRENAL CRISIS

Strategies to prevent adrenal crisis in at-risk individuals include patient education regarding steroid dose adjustments when going through illnesses and stress and medical alert bracelets identifying adrenal insufficiency risk/history.

CLINICS CARE POINTS

- Adrenal insufficiency may present with a chronic and insidious presentation of vague symptoms (anorexia, abdominal/gastrointestinal complaints, weight loss, weakness, and fatigue)
- Adrenal crisis is characterized by refractory hypotension and is a life-threatening medical emergency
- The backbone of treatment for all patients with adrenal insufficiency is glucocorticoid therapy.
- Mineralocorticoid and DHEA replacement may be necessary for patients with primary adrenal insufficiency.

DISCLOSURE

No commercial/financial conflicts of interest.

REFERENCES

1. Kebebew E. Adrenal incidentaloma. N Engl J Med 2021;384(16):1542–51.
2. Reisch N, Peczkowska M, Januszewicz A, et al. Pheochromocytoma: presentation, diagnosis and treatment. J Hypertens 2006 Dec;24(12):2331–9.
3. Vilela LAP, Almeida MQ. Diagnosis and management of primary aldosteronism. Arch Endocrinol Metab 2017 May-Jun;61(3):305–12.
4. Cobb A, Aeddula NR. Primary hyperaldosteronism. Available at:. Treasure Island (FL): StatPearls Publishing; 2023. StatPearls [Internet]. https://www.ncbi.nlm.nih.gov/books/NBK539779/. [Accessed 24 March 2023].
5. Reincke M, Fleseriu M. Cushing Syndrome: A Review. JAMA 2023;330(2):170–81.
6. Petramala L, Olmati F, Concistrè A, et al. Cardiovascular and metabolic risk factors in patients with subclinical Cushing. Endocrine 2020;70:150–63.
7. Czapla-Iskrzycka A, Świątkowska-Stodulska R, Sworczak K. Comorbidities in mild autonomous cortisol secretion - a clinical review of literature. Exp Clin Endocrinol Diabetes 2022;130(9):567–76.
8. Fleseriu M, Auchus R, Bancus I, et al. Consensus on diagnosis and management of Cushing's disease: a guideline update. Lancet Diabetes Endocrinol 2021 Dec; 9(12):847–75.
9. Vaidya A, Hamrahian AH, Bancos I, et al. The evaluation of incidentally discovered adrenal masses. Endocr Pract 2019;25(2):178–92.
10. Fassnacht M, Tsagarakis S, Terzolo M, et al. European Society of Endocrinology clinical practice guidelines on the management of adrenal incidentalomas, in

collaboration with the European Network for the Study of Adrenal Tumors. Eur J Endocrinol 2023 Jul 20;189(1):G1–42.

11. Neary N, Nieman L. Adrenal insufficiency: etiology, diagnosis and treatment. Curr Opin Endocrinol Diabetes Obes 2010;17(3):217–23.

12. Huecker MR, Bhutta BS, Dominique E. Available at:. In: Adrenal insufficiency. Treasure Island (FL): StatPearls Publishing; 2023. StatPearls [Internet]. https://www.ncbi.nlm.nih.gov/books/NBK441832/. [Accessed 17 August 2023].

13. Al-Aridi R, Abdelmannan D, Arafah BM. Biochemical diagnosis of adrenal insufficiency: the added value of dehydroepiandrosterone sulfate measurements. Endocr Pract 2011;17(2):261–70.

14. Bornstein SR, Allolio B, Arlt W, et al. Diagnosis and Treatment of Primary Adrenal Insufficiency: An Endocrine Society Clinical Practice Guideline. J Clin Endocrinol Metabol 2016;101(2):364–89.

15. Flad TM, Conway JD, Cunningham SK, et al. The role of plasma renin activity in evaluating the adequacy of mineralocorticoid replacement in primary adrenal insufficiency. Clin Endocrinol 1996;45(5):529–34.

16. Rushworth RL, Torpy DJ, Falhammar H. Adrenal crisis. N Engl J Med 2019;381(9): 852–61.

Female Reproductive Endocrine Disorders

Monica Selander-Han, DO*, Shelby McGee, DO, Keswick Lo, MD

KEYWORDS

- Primary ovarian insufficiency • Infertility • Osteoporosis • Estrogen • Ovulation
- Amenorrhea • Hormone replacement therapy • Transgender

KEY POINTS

- Normal menstrual cycle is defined as bleeding that lasts for approximately 5 days and cycle intervals of 21 to 35 days.
- It is normal to have a few days of variation between cycle lengths, with more than 10 days of variance being suggestive of anovulation. Heavy menstrual bleeding, or menorrhagia, is defined as blood loss of more than 80 mL; however, the opinion of the patient is used clinically to define abnormally heavy blood loss.
- Polymenorrhea defines menstrual cycles occurring more frequently than every 21 days, while oligomenorrhea defines cycles occurring less often than 35 days.

ABNORMAL UTERINE BLEEDING
Definitions

Normal menstrual cycle is defined as bleeding that lasts for approximately 5 days and cycle intervals of 21 to 35 days. It is normal to have a few days of variation between cycle lengths, with more than 10 days of variance being suggestive of anovulation. Heavy menstrual bleeding, or menorrhagia, is defined as blood loss of more than 80 mL; however, the opinion of the patient is used clinically to define abnormally heavy blood loss. Polymenorrhea defines menstrual cycles occurring more frequently than every 21 days, while oligomenorrhea defines cycles occurring less often than 35 days.[1] Metrorrhagia is the term used for bleeding in between menstrual cycles. There has been debate over the use of these terms, as they are difficult for patients to understand.[2]

Menstruation occurs as a result of a specific and complex hypothalamic–pituitary–ovarian relationship and its effect on the endometrium. The cycle is defined in 2 phases: the earlier phase prior to ovulation and the time following ovulation until the next bleeding begins. The 2 phases are defined based on the endometrial activity and the ovarian activity. Normally, the phase prior to ovulation, referred to as the follicular phase for the ovary or proliferative phase for the endometrium, is mediated by

Department of Family Medicine, Tidelands Health, 4320 Holmestown Road, Myrtle Beach, SC 29588, USA
* Corresponding author.
E-mail address: mselander@tidelandshealth.org

Prim Care Clin Office Pract 51 (2024) 431–443
https://doi.org/10.1016/j.pop.2024.04.002
0095-4543/24/© 2024 Elsevier Inc. All rights reserved.

estrogen-influenced proliferation of the endometrium. During this phase for the ovary, follicles are forming and a dominant follicle is emerging. After ovulation, we enter the secretory (endometrial) and luteal (ovarian) phases, which are dominated by both estrogen and now newly present progesterone, secreted by the corpus luteum cyst which formed when the dominant follicle released the egg. Menstruation occurs from the withdrawal of progesterone when this cyst ceases to function due to lack of beta human chorionic gonadotrophin (bHCG) stimulation.[1]

Alteration of any part of this process results in lack of ovulation and anovulatory bleeding. Without estrogen–progesterone withdrawal, the endometrium continues estrogen-mediated proliferation and has uncoordinated random bleeding and sloughing of different areas of the endometrium. This results in unpredictable, often heavy bleeding.[3]

Etiology

Causes of abnormal uterine bleeding (AUB) have been organized into the following acronym PALM-COEIN. This is supported by International Federation of Gynecology and Obstetrics (FIGO) classification.[1] PALM indicates structural causes of abnormal bleeding while COEIN indicates hormonal or endocrine causes (**Table 1**), and further delineation into ovulatory reasons is shown in **Box 1**.

Anovulation in early puberty, perimenopause, pregnancy, and lactation is considered physiologic.

Evaluation

Evaluation of the patient with AUB starts with a history and physical examination. Screening for blood clotting disorder is necessary to determine if you need to obtain laboratories for abnormalities of hemostasis[4] (**Table 2**).

Physical examination findings suggestive of endocrine causes include hirsutism, acne, obesity, acanthosis nigricans, and thyroid nodules. Also, the physical examination should include a speculum and bimanual examination for the nonadolescent patient to observe for lesions, lacerations, and determine uterine size. This also allows for collection of cervical cancer screening in appropriate populations.[5]

Laboratory evaluation

Initial laboratory evaluation of AUB should include complete blood count (CBC), type and screen, bHCG, thyroid stimulating hormone (TSH), and cervical cancer and chlamydia screening. One should also consider liver function test (LFTs) and iron studies based on clinical correlation. If coagulation screening is positive (see **Table 1**), expand laboratory testing to include Von Willebrand factor antigen, ristocetin cofactor assay, factor VIII, protime/international normalized ratio (PT/INR), prothrombin time (PTT), and fibrinogen.[6]

Table 1 PALM-COEIN			
P	Polyp	C	Coagulopathy
A	Adenomyosis	O	Ovulatory
L	Leiomyoma	E	Endometrial
M	Malignancy/hyperplasia	I	Iatrogenic
		N	Not classified

Box 1
Causes of abnormal uterine bleeding-O

Hyperandrogenism (PCOS, congenital adrenal hyperplasia, androgen-secreting tumor)

Hypothalamic (anorexia nervosa)

Hyperprolactinemia

Thyroid disorders

Primary pituitary disorder

Premature ovarian failure

Iatrogenic (radiation, chemotherapy)

Medications (birth control pills, blood thinners, chemotherapy)

Imaging

First-line imaging consists of transvaginal ultrasonography. Alternative options include saline infused sonohysterogram, which is more accurate at determining intracavitary pathology and pelvic MRI.[5]

Endometrial sampling

Endometrial biopsy is indicated as first-line evaluation for patients aged over 45 years but can be considered for patients under the age of 45 years if the following exist: obesity, nulliparous, hypertensive, known polycystic ovarian syndrome (PCOS), failed medical management, persistent AUB.[7]

Treatment

Goals of therapy

Therapeutic options are directed at the goals of the patient. Most often these include stopping current bleeding, prevention of further bothersome bleeding, preventing anemia, contraception, and reducing risk of hyperplasia. In the case where a pregnancy is desired, management is different and out of the scope of this article.[8]

Treatment will first be directed at any identified underlying cause, such as management of hyper or hypothyroidism and treatment of pituitary tumor. After all underlying causes have been identified and treated, other medical treatment options can be considered (**Table 3**).

Generally, abnormal Uterine bleeding - ovulatory (AUB-O) can be treated medically and surgery is not indicated. If the patient has completed childbearing and declines medical management, or medical management fails or is not tolerated, hysterectomy is a surgical option. Although hysterectomy has been shown in some studies to give

---

Table 2
Historical markers of possible clotting disorder

Any One of the Following	Any Two of the Following
Heavy menses since menarche	Bruising frequently
Postpartum hemorrhage	Epistaxis
Bleeding associated with surgery	Gum bleeding
Bleeding associated with dental work	Family history

Table 3 Treatment options for AUB	
Progesterone Only	**Combination Estrogen and Progesterone**
Levonorgestrel intra-uterine device (IUD) (appropriate for all ages)	Oral contraceptive pills
Megestrol acetate	Transdermal patch
Norethindrone	Vaginal ring
Medroxyprogesterone acetate	
Depot medroxyprogesterone acetate	

improved results over medical options, it has also been demonstrated to have equal efficacy to the levonorgestrel IUD.[9]Coexistence of structural causes such as polyps is another indication for surgical treatment.

Uterine ablation is not a first-line treatment of AUB-O, and thorough counseling is necessary.[10]

Summary

In summary, AUB is defined with menorrhagia, polymenorrhea, and menorrhagia. Menstruation is the effect on the endometrium by the hypothalamic–pituitary–ovarian axis. Causes for AUB can be organized by using the acronym PALM-COEIN but other pathologic causes can include thyroid disorders, pituitary disorders, and medications. Evaluation includes a thorough history and physical examination as well as laboratory evaluation to include testing for coagulopathies.

PRIMARY OVARIAN INSUFFICIENCY
Introduction

Primary ovarian insufficiency (POI), also known as premature ovarian failure, hypergonadotropic hypogonadism, or early menopause, is a troubling diagnosis to give a young woman. Often, the cause of ovarian failure may be idiopathic. Goals of care include managing their symptoms (hot flashes, vaginal dryness, and mood changes) and giving them the proper counseling on how to prevent health issues caused by decreased estrogen levels.

Clinical Presentation and Diagnosis

Primary ovarian failure is defined as the development of hypergonadotropic hypogonadism before 40 years of age. It is important to ensure that the symptoms cannot be attributed to the use of oral contraceptives. Pertinent laboratories to order include beta-hCG, TSH, prolactin, follicle-stimulating hormone, and estradiol. If a patient is menstruating, estradiol must be obtained on day 3 of the cycle.[11]

An easy interpretation of these laboratories includes the following:

1. Abnormal TSH, beta-hCG, or prolactin rules out POS as a primary differential
2. If FSH and estradiol are high: Pituitary adenoma versus midcycle surge
3. If FSH and estradiol are low: Repeat laboratories, then POI versus hypogonadotropic hypogonadism
4. If FSH is high and estradiol is borderline low: Repeat laboratories

Some factors that distinguish POI from other conditions are hot flashes, night sweats, insomnia, inability to conceive, and elevated FSH. The presence of any of these symptoms, along with FSH levels greater than 25 to 40 on 2 consecutive months, lead to a diagnosis after other causes of amenorrhea (pregnancy, thyroid disease, and hypothalamic/pituitary dysfunction) have been ruled out.[12]

Laboratory tests to consider for an amenorrhea workup are as following: B-hGC, FSH, TSH, testosterone, estradiol, prolactin, dehydroepiandrosterone-sulfate (DHEAS), 17-hydroxyprogesterone (17-OH-P), autoimmune workup, and karyotype analysis.[13] In addition to these laboratories, a pelvic ultrasound and karyotype analysis can be performed.[14] Other supportive diagnostic considerations that can be obtained are chromosome analysis, array comparative genomic hybridization (CGH), and family analysis.[12]

It is not common practice to investigate genetic causes of POI.[15] However, the prevalence of the genetic-associated POI is approximately 20% to 25%. One of the most common genetic causes of POI is Turner syndrome. This caused a reduction in the ovarian reserve and primordial follicle atresia.[12] The following genes are associated with POI: NR5A1, NOBOX, FIGLA, and FOXL2. Genetic mutations to the FSH or LH receptors, inhibin A, GDF9, or BMP15 can also contribute to the condition.[15]

Treatments and Prevention

While there is no cure or known agent to slow the progression of POI, there are treatments available for symptoms that coincide with low levels of estrogen. Estrogen/progestin pills can be utilized in this condition for a variety of reasons. Commonly, they are used for relief of hot flashes, night sweats, vaginal dryness, and bone loss prevention. Other agents that can be administered for hot flashes are venlafaxine XR, paroxetine, clonidine, and fezolinetant.[13] Alternative options are cognitive behavioral therapy, oxybutynin, or gabapentin.[16] Ospemifene or vaginal estradiol cream can be used for moderate-to-severe vaginal dryness.

Patients should be educated about the increased risk of diabetes and osteoporosis with POI. There is a 12% higher risk of developing diabetes in patients with POI.[16] Early interventions including healthy eating and improving exercise habits can prevent the development of diabetes, especially in those with obesity syndrome or a family history of diabetes.[15] Patients with POI are also at higher risk of osteoporosis and should take 1200 mg of elemental calcium daily and 800 to 1000 IU of vitamin D daily if serum 25-hydroxyvitamin D is below 30 ng/ml.[14]

COMPLICATIONS

POI affects a woman's physical and emotional well-being. Other associated endocrine deficiencies, as well as anxiety, depression, or both, may develop. Women with POI have a higher risk of developing metabolic disease or having reduced bone mineral density which can be avoided with early screening and education. Spontaneous remission with conception is another complication that occurs in less than 10% of patients.[14] Thus, there is a risk when starting patients on certain medicines that are teratogenic or may affect the fetus.

SUMMARY

While there is no cure for POI, there are treatments that can ameliorate symptoms and options for family planning such as adoption and embryo donation. It is important to provide support and comfort when disclosing the diagnosis with patients and to address the emotional distress they may experience when processing the news.

Primary care providers should screen for and treat metabolic disease and osteoporosis in patients with POI. Because osteoporosis is more likely to develop in this population, they should be encouraged to begin weight-bearing exercises, take 1200 mg of calcium daily and have their a fracture risk assessment tool to determine the patient's probability of sustaining a bone fracture (frax score) and vitamin D levels monitored.[14]

TRANSGENDER
Introduction

"Transgender" is a term to describe people who express themselves as a different gender from their assigned birth sex. It is not to be confused with the terms "intersex," "transvestite," or "transexual." Intersex individuals were born with genetic, hormonal, and/or physical characteristics that vary from the binary definitions and terminology used to label a person male or female. Transvestism is different from transgender because the person will dress like the opposite gender, but does not necessarily identify with that gender. This term should not be used as it can be considered disrespectful.[17,18] "Transexual" is a historic term that relates to a transgender person seeking body and hormonal modification to affirm their gender.[18,19]

Transgender patients may or may not suffer with gender dysphoria. For those who do, gender-affirming medical care can be available to them if they meet eligibility criteria.[17] Here, we discuss the current recommendations and medical treatment options for the transgender population.

Clinical Presentation and Diagnosis

A transgender patient may openly express their desired gender or they may be exploring their thoughts and feelings about undergoing the transition. If a patient reports that they do not belong in the body of the sex they were born and desire to be the other sex or a different gender, it is likely they are experiencing gender incongruence.[20] A prepubertal patient will have increased distress at the onset of puberty. An adult transgender patient may present requesting hormone treatments or a referral for surgery to modify their body to obtain more feminine or masculine features.[20] Gender incongruence or gender dysphoria can be diagnosed using the criteria listed in the Diagnostic and Statistical Manueal of Mental Disorders (5th edition) (DSM-5).

Physicians should do a good physical examination, making sure to also take note of their current sexual characteristics using the Tanner stage[17] (**Table 4**). A thorough

Table 4 Tanner stages 1 to 5	
1	• No pubic hair, breast or scrotal growth
2	• Breast: palpable areolar bud • Pubic hair: sparse and straight • Scrotum: enlargement
3	• Breast: peripheral bud development • Pubic hair: more follicles, curly • Penis: grows in length
4	• Breast: enlargement and elevation of areolas forming a "secondary mound" • Pubic hair: spares the thighs, dark, coarse and curly • Penis/scrotum/testes: continues to grow
5	• Breast: adult size with even contour • Pubic hair: growth on genitals and thighs • Penis/scrotum: adult size

psych evaluation must also be done, keeping an open mind as to what could cause their psychiatric changes beyond gender incongruence. The extent and consistency of their challenges with gender dysphoria should also be reviewed and documented.[18]

Treatments

General
Gender-affirming hormone therapies should be withheld until the patient is evaluated by a psychiatrist who is knowledgeable about the criteria for diagnosing and treating gender dysphoric/incongruent individuals. The Endocrine Society believes patients may have sufficient mental capacity to understand the permanent outcomes of hormone treatment by 16 years.[17] It is discouraged to begin testosterone or estrogen therapy until this age, but at 16 years, hormone therapy can begin as long as the patient continues to have gender dysphoria/incongruence and has reached Tanner stage 2 after puberty has begun.[19] Patients should clearly be informed of the potential for permanent loss of fertility.[20] Other risks include polycythemia, transaminitis, hypertension, hyperlipidemia, cardiovascular disease, and breast cancer (for trans men) and thrombosis, transaminitis, hyperprolactinemia, and breast cancer (for trans women).[20]

Mental health
Emotional support should always be offered and available for these individuals as they have a higher risk of developing depression and a higher rate of suicide compared to the rest of the population. In fact, more than 40% of transindividuals have attempted suicide.[20] Perform routine screenings for depression, anxiety, substance use, self-injury, bullying, homelessness, and suicidality.[18]

Puberty suppression
GnRH agonists, such as histrelin and leuprolide, are the most common agents used to slow or stop the development of secondary sex characteristics by suppressing the hypothalamic–pituitary–gonadal axis while teens explore their gender identity until they are ready to begin gender-affirming hormone therapy. Children at the age of 8 to 14 years can start gondotrophin releasing hormone (GnRH) agonists to delay deepening of the voice or the development of facial hair, Adam's apple or breast tissue as mentioned earlier.[17] If menses, erections, or progressive hair growth are present, the dose can be increased.[19] The Endocrine Society recommends measuring a baseline height, weight, blood pressure, and tanner stage 2 to 4 times a year while taking these medications as well as biannual testosterone levels (for patients with testes) or FSH, LH, and estradiol levels (for patients with ovaries).[17,18] They also recommend ordering a dual X-ray absorptiometry (DEXA) scan before starting treatment and annually thereafter.[17]

Once the induction of puberty begins, the examiner should record a baseline height, weight, blood pressure, and tanner stage. These measurements should be taken every 3 to 6 months until 25 to 30 years of age. Bone mineral density should also be monitored annually during that time using a DEXA scan. Transgender male individuals should get the following laboratories once or twice a year: hemoglobin, hematocrit, lipids, testosterone, and 25-hydroxyvitamin D. Transgender female individuals should get the following laboratories once or twice a year: prolactin, estradiol, and 25-hydroxyvitamin D.[17]

Hormone therapy: Transgender female individuals
Estradiol is the hormone of choice for transgender female individuals. The dose should be increased gradually with 200 pg/mL as the goal serum estradiol level.[20] Serum

estrogen, serum testosterone levels, and a basic metabolic panel should be reviewed quarterly and then biannually after the first year.[18]

Hormone therapy: Transgender male individuals

Testosterone is the hormone of choice for transgender male individuals. The goal serum testosterone level ranges from 400 to 700 ng/dL.[17] Testosterone and hematocrit levels must be checked before starting treatment, as well as quarterly for the first year. They can be ordered biannually after 12 months. Prolactin levels should be reviewed before starting and then yearly.[18]

Surgery

Surgical treatment options that are available, but not necessarily always performed are chest reconstruction, hysterectomy, phalloplasty, and erectile prosthesis. The endocrine society does not recommend these surgeries until at least 18 years of age.[17]

Summary

In summary, there are a variety of ways to support transgender patients. It is important to provide a comfortable, unbiased atmosphere so they will seek medical help or health screenings when they need it. Allowing them to make decisions about their body and appearance helps to close the gap in care that they have experienced historically.

MENOPAUSE

Introduction

Menopause is a retrospective diagnosis and is defined as the cessation of menstrual activity for 12 consecutive months without any other pathologic or physiologic cause. Although the average age of menopause occurs at 51.4 years, menopausal transition begins on average at 47 years.[21] This occurs as a result of ovarian follicle depletion, resulting in endocrinologic changes marked by decreasing estradiol and increasing follicle-stimulating hormone. Multiple factors can affect the timing of menopause, which include sociodemographic differences, lower parity, lower socioeconomic status, and tobacco use.[22] Lifestyle changes and medications can be used for management of symptoms. In those women with severe symptoms, considering benefit–risk ratio, they may be a candidate for hormonal replacement therapies.

Clinical Presentation and Diagnosis

While diagnosis of menopause is retrospective, consideration of menopausal transition in women is correlated with age and is determined by changes in menstrual interval, with or without menopausal symptoms. In women over the age of 45 years, diagnosis is made clinically as 12 months of amenorrhea in the absence of other pathologic or physiologic causes. Early menopause may be considered in women aged 40 to 45 years, but other causes of menstrual cycle dysfunction must be ruled out. For those aged under 40 years with intermenstrual changes or menopausallike symptoms should be evaluated for POI as discussed elsewhere in this article. Over 80% of women will experience 1 or more symptoms, these are often nonspecific but commonly include[22–24]

- Vasomotor symptoms—commonly described as "hot flashes," the most common symptomatic complaint that occurs in up to 80% of women[23]
- Changes in mood—increased risk of depression compared to premenopausal years[24]

- Sleep disturbance—often secondary to hot flashes, may also be due to associated depression/anxiety
- Vulvovaginal atrophy—can lead to decreased vaginal lubrication and sexual dysfunction

In women over the age of 45 years, diagnosis is made by clinical assessment; FSH does not need to be measured. In fact, FSH concentrations in perimenopausal women can be variable and are not a reliable marker for diagnosis.[25] Pregnancy should always be considered in all sexually active women with amenorrhea who are not using reliable contraception; therefore, serum hCG should be obtained to rule it out.

TREATMENTS

Management of perimenopause is typically by acute management of symptoms with pharmacologic treatment. Lifestyle modifications such as maintain healthy weight, increasing exercise, cooling management of body temperature, and avoiding triggers such as alcohol or spicy foods can be considered. However, evidence suggesting these adjustments improve menopausal symptoms is limited and mixed.[26] Menopausal hormone therapy (MHT) remains the most effective means of treatment, particularly for vasomotor symptoms and genitourinary syndrome of menopause (vulvovaginal atrophy). This includes both systemic and topical/vaginal replacement of estrogen. Contraindications include history of breast or endometrial cancer, previous stroke or venous thromboembolic event, active liver disease, unexplained vaginal bleeding, or transient ischemic attack. There are multiple formulations with different delivery methods of hormone therapy[27].

- Oral estrogen, transdermal estrogen, and topical estradiol are effective in treating vasomotor symptoms.
- Low-dose vaginal estrogen is often used for management of vulvovaginal atrophy.
  - Like other systemic estrogen preparations, high-dose vaginal estrogen can be used to treat vasomotor symptoms.
    - When initiating estrogen therapy, progestin should be prescribed to women with an intact uterus to prevent endometrial hyperplasia as estrogen treatment alone can increase this. It is not necessary to prescribe progestin to those who have undergone hysterectomy given the lack of uterus; thus, there will no longer be a concern for developing endometrial hyperplasia and carcinoma.[28]

Table 5
Management of perimenopausal symptoms

Oral Estrogen Transdermal estrogen Topical estrogen	Moderate-to-severe vasomotor symptoms (hot flashes)	Add progestin therapy to patients with intact uterus
SSRI/SNRI	Menopausal-related depression Vasomotor symptoms	Venlafaxine and paroxetine shown to be more efficacious in some studies
Gabapentin	Vasomotor symptoms	
Black cohosh Isoflavone/phytoestrogen (plant-based supplements)	Vasomotor symptoms	Efficacy not well established

There are also nonhormonal pharmacologic agents; these have varying degrees of effectiveness but may be considered in women who are not candidates of hormonal therapy or who prefer to avoid MHT due to concern of adverse effects and complications and further explanation given in **Table 5**.

- Selective serotonin reuptake inhibitor (SSRIs)/Serotonin and norepinephrine reuptake inhibitors (SNRIs) can be used to treat menopausal-related depression.
  - These may also help to relieve vasomotor symptoms.[29,30] In clinical studies, some SSRI/SNRIs were shown to be more effective than others at relieving symptoms, notably venlafaxine and paroxetine.[30]
- Gabapentin has also shown to be effective for hot flashes in some women.[31]
- The use of supplements and other alternative therapies are common among postmenopausal women. However, their safety and efficacy are not well established.[32]

COMPLICATIONS

There are many long-term effects attributable to estrogen deficiency. Women will begin to have bone mineral density loss in the perimenopausal phase, leading to increased risk of fracture at the postmenopausal age. Menopause may also result in an increased risk of cardiovascular disease. Lipid changes with increases in low-density lipoprotein and total cholesterol have been seen, particularly in late-stage perimenopause and early postmenopause.[32] There is also some evidence that suggest estrogen helps to preserve cognitive function in women without dementia. However, estrogen replacement therapy has not shown to provide global cognitive benefits.[33]

SUMMARY

Menopause is a natural process that women experience as they age. Medications and lifestyle changes can be beneficial to combat bothersome symptoms such as hot flashes, insomnia, vaginal dryness, and mood changes. In primary care, it is important to counsel young women about cardiovascular health, healthy diets, and avoiding tobacco use to avoid complications with heart disease, diabetes, or osteoporosis after menopause begins.

CLINICS CARE POINTS

- A strong suspicion of POI should be held when female individuals under 40 years have hot flashes with menstrual irregularities.
- Hormone therapy is used to manage vasomotor symptoms, vaginal atrophy, and fractures.
- POI is one of the four most common causes of secondary amenorrhea. Other more common causes are polycystic ovary syndrome, hyperprolactinemia, and hypothalamic amenorrhea.
- Puberty suppression should not begin until the child has reached Tanner stage 2 and gender-affirming hormone therapy should not begin until after puberty.
- Mental health issues, substance abuse, and suicide rates are higher in the transgender population than in cisgender individuals.
- The Endocrine Society recommends a psychiatric evaluation when patients are requesting gender-affirming hormone therapy.

- The standard of care at this time is to allow transgender patients to freely express themselves based on what makes them comfortable. It is unethical to try changing them to identify with their sex assigned at birth.
- The average age of menopause is 51.4 years. Starting menopause below age 45 years is considered "early" and starting after age 55 years is considered "late."
- Complications of menopause include bone mineral density loss and increased risk for cardiovascular disease. Many women also experience a decreased quality of life as a result of menopausal symptoms.

DISCLOSURE

The authors have nothing to disclose.

REFERENCES

1. Munro MG, Critchley HO, Broder MS, et al, FIGO Working Group on Menstrual Disorders. FIGO classification system (PALM-COEIN) for causes of abnormal uterine bleeding in nongravid women of reproductive age. FIGO Working Group on Menstrual Disorders. Int J Gynaecol Obstet 2011;113:3–13.
2. Fraser IS, Critchley HO, Munro MG, et al, Writing Group for this Menstrual Agreement Process. A process designed to lead to international agreement on terminologies and definitions used to describe abnormalities of menstrual bleeding. Writing Group for this Menstrual Agreement Process. Fertil Steril 2007;87: 466–76 [published erratum appears in Fertil Steril 2007;88:538].
3. Jones K, Sung S. Anovulatory bleeding. In: StatPearls [internet]. Treasure Island (FL): StatPearls Publishing; 2024 Jan. Available at: https://www.ncbi.nlm.nih.gov/books/NBK549773.
4. Von Willebrand disease in women. ACOG Committee Opinion No. 451. American College of Obstetricians and Gynecologists. Obstet Gynecol 2009;114:1439–43.
5. National Guideline Alliance (UK). Evidence reviews for diagnostic test accuracy in investigation for women presenting with heavy menstrual bleeding: heavy menstrual bleeding (update): evidence review A. London: National Institute for Health and Care Excellence (NICE); 2018 (NICE Guideline, No. 88.) Diagnosis of heavy menstrual bleeding. Available at: https://www.ncbi.nlm.nih.gov/books/NBK569003/.
6. Kouides PA, Conard J, Peyvandi F, et al. Hemostasis and menstruation: appropriate investigation for underlying disorders of hemostasis in women with excessive menstrual bleeding. Fertil Steril 2005;84(5):1345–51.
7. Hysteroscopy. Technology Assessment No. 7. American College of Obstetricians and Gynecologists. Obstet Gynecol 2011;117:1486–91.
8. National Guideline Alliance (UK). Evidence reviews for management of heavy menstrual bleeding: heavy menstrual bleeding (update): evidence review B. London: National Institute for Health and Care Excellence (NICE); 2018 Mar (NICE Guideline, No. 88.) Available at: https://www.ncbi.nlm.nih.gov/books/NBK569015/.
9. Hurskainen R, Teperi J, Rissanen P, et al. Quality of life and cost-effectiveness of levonorgestrel-releasing intrauterine system versus hysterectomy for treatment of menorrhagia: a randomised trial. Lancet 2001;357:273.
10. Ang WC, Hickey M. Postmenopausal bleeding after endometrial ablation: where are we now? Maturitas 2011;69:195–6.
11. Chen M, Jiang H, Zhang C. Selected genetic factors associated with primary ovarian insufficiency. Int J Mol Sci 2023;24(5):4423.

12. Schorge JO, Schaffer JI, Cunningham G, et al. Williams' gynecology. New York, NY: McGraw-Hill Medical; 2008.
13. Nelson LM. Clinical practice. primary ovarian insufficiency. N Engl J Med 2009; 360(6):606–14.
14. Ishizuka B. Current understanding of the etiology, symptomatology, and treatment options in premature ovarian insufficiency (POI). Front Endocrinol 2021; 12:626924.
15. The 2023 Nonhormone Therapy Position Statement of The North American Menopause Society Advisory Panel. The 2023 nonhormone therapy position statement of The North American Menopause Society. Menopause 2023;30(6):573–90.
16. Lambrinoudaki I, Paschou SA. Hormone therapy for menopause and premature ovarian insufficiency. Best Pract Res Clin Endocrinol Metab 2021;35(6):101597.
17. Salas-Humara C, Sequeira GM, Rossi W, et al. Gender affirming medical care of transgender youth. Curr Probl Pediatr Adolesc Health Care 2019;49(9):100683.
18. Klein DA, Paradise SL, Goodwin ET. Caring for transgender and gender-diverse persons: what clinicians should know. Am Fam Physician 2018;98(11):645–53.
19. Hembree WC, Cohen-Kettenis PT, Gooren L, et al. Endocrine treatment of gender-dysphoric/gender-incongruent persons: an endocrine society clinical practice guideline. J Clin Endocrinol Metab 2017;102(11):3869–903 [published correction appears in j clin endocrinol metab. 2018 Feb 1;103(2):699] [published correction appears in J Clin Endocrinol Metab. 2018 Jul 1;103(7):2758-2759].
20. Radix A. Hormone therapy for transgender adults. Urol Clin North Am 2019;46(4): 467–73.
21. McKinlay SM, Brambilla DJ, Posner JG. The normal menopause transition. Maturitas 1992 Jan;14(2):103–15.
22. Gold EB. The timing of the age at which natural menopause occurs. Obstet Gynecol Clin North Am 2011;38(3):425–40.
23. Woods NF, Mitchell ES. Symptoms during the perimenopause: prevalence, severity, trajectory, and significance in women's lives. Am J Med 2005 Dec 19; 118(Suppl 12B):14–24.
24. Bromberger JT, Meyer PM, Kravitz HM, et al. Psychologic distress and natural menopause: a multiethnic community study. Am J Publ Health 2001 Sep;91(9): 1435–42.
25. Hee J, MacNaughton J, Bangah M, et al. Perimenopausal patterns of gonadotrophins, immunoreactive inhibin, oestradiol and progesterone. Maturitas 1993 Dec; 18(1):9–20.
26. "The 2023 Nonhormone Therapy Position Statement of The North American Menopause Society" Advisory Panel. "The 2023 nonhormone therapy position statement of the north american menopause society" advisory panel. the 2023 nonhormone therapy position statement of the north american menopause society. Menopause 2023 Jun 1;30(6):573–90. https://doi.org/10.1097/GME.0000000000002200.
27. Stuenkel CA, Davis SR, Gompel A, et al. Treatment of symptoms of the menopause: an endocrine society clinical practice guideline. J Clin Endocrinol Metab 2015 Nov;100(11):3975–4011.
28. Barrett-Connor E, Slone S, Greendale G, et al. The postmenopausal estrogen/progestin interventions study: primary outcomes in adherent women. Maturitas 1997 Jul;27(3):261–74.
29. Loprinzi CL, Barton DL, Sloan JA, et al. Mayo clinic and north central cancer treatment group hot flash studies: a 20-year experience. Menopause 2008 Jul-Aug;15(4 Pt 1):655–60.

30. Loprinzi CL, Sloan J, Stearns V, et al. Newer antidepressants and gabapentin for hot flashes: an individual patient pooled analysis. J Clin Oncol 2009;27(17): 2831–7.
31. Derby CA, Crawford SL, Pasternak RC, et al. Lipid changes during the menopause transition in relation to age and weight: the study of women's health across the nation. Am J Epidemiol 2009;169(11):1352–61.
32. Keenan NL, Mark S, Fugh-Berman A, et al. Severity of menopausal symptoms and use of both conventional and complementary/alternative therapies. Menopause 2003 Nov-Dec;10(6):507–15.
33. Shumaker SA, Legault C, Rapp SR, et al, WHIMS Investigators. Estrogen plus progestin and the incidence of dementia and mild cognitive impairment in postmenopausal women: the Women's Health Initiative Memory Study: a randomized controlled trial. JAMA 2003 May 28;289(20):2651–62.

Metabolic Bone Disease

LaRae L. Seemann, MD[a], Christina T. Hanos, MD[a],
George G.A. Pujalte, MD[a,b],*

KEYWORDS

- Bone metabolism • Metabolic bone disease • Osteomalacia • Osteoporosis
- Paget disease • Primary hyperparathyroidism • Rickets

KEY POINTS

- Osteoporosis is the most common metabolic bone disease; 1 in 3 women and 1 in 5 men aged 50 years or older will encounter osteoporotic fractures during their lifetime.
- Vitamin D deficiency impairs absorption of calcium and phosphorus, and thus, can lead to osteomalacia. Clinicians should identify patients at risk for vitamin D deficiency.
- Bone pain, joint pain, and skeletal deformities should prompt a workup for metabolic bone disease, especially in the presence of other risk factors.
- Endocrine disturbances such as hyperparathyroidism, hyperthyroidism, and hypogonadism can negatively impact the skeletal system.

INTRODUCTION

Metabolic bone disease (MBD) encompasses a group of disorders characterized by abnormalities in bone metabolism, structure, or mineralization. Bones are dynamic structures undergoing a daily process of formation and resorption, such that the adult skeleton is replaced roughly every 10 years.[1] When this equilibrium is disrupted, MBDs can manifest, leading to various skeletal abnormalities and increased susceptibility to fractures.

Bones form through a process known as ossification, which occurs in 2 ways: intramembranous ossification and endochondral ossification. Intramembranous ossification involves direct mineralization of mesenchymal (undifferentiated) connective tissue, leading to the formation of flat bones, such as those in the skull. On the other hand, endochondral ossification starts with a cartilage model that gradually transforms into bone tissue[2] and is the process responsible for the formation of most bones in the body, including long bones like the femur and the humerus. During both types of

©2024 Mayo Foundation for Medical Education and Research.

[a] Department of Family Medicine, Mayo Clinic, 4500 San Pablo Road, Jacksonville, FL 32224, USA; [b] Department of Orthopedic Surgery, Mayo Clinic, 4500 San Pablo Road, Jacksonville, FL 32224, USA
* Corresponding author.
E-mail address: Pujalate.George@mayo.edu

Prim Care Clin Office Pract 51 (2024) 445–454
https://doi.org/10.1016/j.pop.2024.04.005   **primarycare.theclinics.com**

ossification, osteoblasts play a crucial role in secreting bone matrix composed of collagen and noncollagenous organic materials.[1,2] This matrix later undergoes mineralization through deposition of calcium and phosphate ions onto collagen fibers within the developing bone, thus forming mature, hard bone tissue.[1,2] Adequate levels of calcium and phosphate in the body are crucial for maintaining proper bone mineralization and overall bone health. Vitamin D is a major regulator of calcium and phosphate in the blood, promoting its absorption from the intestines, reabsorption in the kidneys, and mobilization from bone tissue.[3]

DISCUSSION
Osteoporosis

Background and prevalence
The most common MBD is osteoporosis, characterized by low total bone mass, microarchitectural bone disruption, and skeletal fragility, resulting in decreased bone strength and increased risk of fractures.[4] As the global population ages and life expectancy rises, osteoporosis is emerging as a widespread epidemic. Presently, over 200 million individuals are estimated to be affected by osteoporosis, including approximately 10 million Americans.[5,6] Recent data from the International Osteoporosis Foundation reveal that globally, 1 in 3 women and 1 in 5 men aged 50 years or older will encounter osteoporotic fractures during their lifetime.[6,7] It is important to note that individuals may also develop secondary osteoporosis from comorbid disease or medications, most notably, glucocorticoids.[8] Androgen-deprivation therapy for prostate cancer places men at increased risk of osteoporosis.[9] The high prevalence of disease is due to a multitude of risk factors that contribute to disease development along with its insidious progression, with osteoporotic fracture often being the first sign. Using screening tools to stratify patients at higher risk and identify underlying or imminent bone disease is critical.

Evaluation
Bone mineral density (BMD) determined by dual-energy X-ray absorptiometry is the standard measure for the diagnosis osteoporosis and assessment of fracture risk. BMD is recognized as both fixed and modifiable. Fixed risk factors include age, height loss, family history, female sex, ethnicity, previous fracture, and estrogen deficiency as seen in postmenopausal women and those with amenorrhea.[5–7,10,11] Modifiable risk factors that impact bone directly, as well as increased risk of fracture independently, include smoking, body mass index less than 20 kg/m^2, alcohol use greater than 2 standard drinks per day, malnutrition with low dietary calcium intake, vitamin D deficiency, eating disorders, frequent falls, and insufficient exercise.[3,4,12,13] The Fracture Risk Assessment Tool (FRAX) serves as a predictive tool for assessing fractures based on clinical risk factors, with or without incorporating femoral neck BMD. BMD testing should be performed in women aged 65 years or older, men aged 70 years or older, and postmenopausal women and men older than 50 years of age based on risk factor profile.[12–15] Additionally, vertebral imaging should be performed on certain men and women based on their BMD T-scores at the spine, total hip, or femoral neck.[12–14] Diagnostic criteria for osteoporosis based on T-score interpretation are illustrated in **Table 1**. Medical management of osteoporosis is recommended for individuals with low BMD (T-score of −1.0 to −2.5) and a 10 year risk of hip fracture of 3% or greater or 10 year risk of a major osteoporosis-related fracture of 20% or greater, as determined by FRAX assessment.[16]

A fragility fracture is a pathologic fracture that results from minimal trauma, such as a fall from standing height or no identifiable trauma at all. This type of fracture is a sign

Table 1	
Diagnostic criteria for osteoporosis	
Classification	**T-Score**
Normal	−1.0 or higher
Osteopenia	−1.0 to −2.5
Osteoporosis	−2.5 or lower

Data from Cosman F, de Beur SJ, LeBoff MS, et al. Clinician's Guide to Prevention and Treatment of Osteoporosis. Osteoporos Int. 2014;25:2359-2381 [Cosman F, de Beur SJ, LeBoff MS, et al. Erratum to: Clinician's guide to prevention and treatment of osteoporosis. Osteoporos Int. 2015;26:2045-2047].

of osteoporosis but may also be a symptom in patients with known osteoporosis. Fragility fracture is consider a major risk factor for osteoporosis, and if T-score is below −2.5 SD with simultaneous fragility fracture, the patient meets criteria for severe osteoporosis. Typical fracture sites of fragility fractures include vertebral, proximal femur, distal forearm, and proximal humerus, mostly due to their loadbearing nature.

Management

Although the FRAX tool is useful for predicting the 10 year probability of hip fracture and other major osteoporotic fracture, the tool does have limitations. It is not validated for use with total hip or lumbar spine BMD, ethnic minorities, individuals already receiving treatment, or patients younger than 40 years or older than 90 years of age.[17] Clinicians should also consider fall history as this risk factor is not included in risk calculation. The goal of treating osteoporosis is to reduce the risk of fractures.

Pharmacologic management of osteoporosis consists of antiresorptive agents (eg, bisphosphonates, denosumab), hormonal therapies (eg, selective estrogen receptor modulators, estrogen-progestin therapy, testosterone therapy, calcitonin, and parathyroid hormone analogues), and emerging therapies in investigative stages (eg, humanized monoclonal antibodies and selective cathepsin K inhibitors).[18] First-line drugs for patients at high risk of fracture include alendronate, risedronate, zoledronic acid, and denosumab.

Bisphosphonates (eg, alendronate, risedronate, ibandronate) are available in various formulations, with most using extended interval dosing. Rare adverse effects of bisphosphonates include osteonecrosis of the jaw and low-trauma atypical femur fractures.[18] Bisphosphonates accumulate in bone and continue to be released for years after treatment cessation, so drug holidays can be considered 3 to 5 years after initiation for patients at moderate fracture risk and 6 to 10 years after initiation for patients at higher fracture risk. The evidence is unclear on when to restart osteoporotic treatment after a drug holiday, but substantial BMD loss or a fracture are potential reasons to resume therapy.[19]

Denosumab is a monoclonal antibody that inhibits receptor activator of nuclear factor $\kappa\beta$ to decrease bone resorption. Denosumab can cause hypocalcemia, so calcium levels should be corrected prior to initiating treatment. This medication may also cause osteonecrosis of the jaw in up to 6.6% of patients. A drug holiday is not recommended as cessation is associated with a decrease in BMD after 2 years. If denosumab is discontinued, bisphosphonates are effective after short-term therapy but less so after longer term therapy. Nevertheless, after 2 or more years of denosumab therapy, all patient should receive either zolendronate or alendronate if therapy is discontinued. [20]

Selective estrogen receptor modulators, such as raloxifene, are first-line therapy for patients requiring reduced risk of spine fracture only and should be considered in women at risk of developing breast cancer as it has selective antagonistic effects on breast tissue. Raloxifene may also be used during a drug holiday from a bisphosphonate if weaker antiresorptive therapy is needed.[20] Hormonal therapy with estrogens or estrogen–progestin can be considered in high-risk postmenopausal women if other treatments have been deemed inappropriate or the patient has severe vasomotor symptoms. Testosterone therapy is recommended exclusively for men at high risk of osteoporotic fracture and whose testosterone levels are less than 200 ng/dL.[15]

Calcitonin is a synthetic polypeptide hormone approved for women who have been postmenopausal for more than 5 years when alternative drugs are not feasible, mostly because data do not demonstrate a reduction in nonverterbral fractures.[21] Parathyroid hormone analogues, teriparatide and abaloparatide, are anabolic and stimulate osteoblast activity. Duration of therapy for these is limited to 2 years due to development of osteosarcoma in rats, and this class of medication should be avoided altogether if the patient has preexisting hypercalcemia. Other promising investigational drugs include romosozumab, a humanized monoclonal antibody that inhibits sclerostin, and odanacatib, a selective inhibitor of cathepsin K.

There is clinical controversy over the follow-up interval for monitoring BMD once treatment is initiated due to a lack of consistent evidence from randomized clinical trials. The National Osteoporosis Foundation recommends monitoring BMD every 1 to 2 years after treatment initiation and every 2 years thereafter.[13] The North American Menopause Society noted that repeat testing in women receiving osteoporosis therapy may not be clinically useful until at least 1 to 2 years after initiating treatment.[22] However, other studies suggest a 4 year interval is appropriate.[12,13,23,24]

Osteomalacia

Background and prevalence

In contrast to osteoporosis, osteomalacia is an impairment of bone composition rather than bone mass. Pathophysiology stems from either a deficiency in bone substrate elements (eg, calcium and phosphate), excessive inhibition of mineralization, or insufficient or ineffective mineralization factors (eg, vitamin D), all of which result in accumulation of unmineralized matrix in the skeleton, and thus soft bones.[25,26] Clinical features of osteomalacia include musculoskeletal pain, skeletal deformity, muscle weakness, and symptomatic hypocalcemia (eg, muscle cramps, paresthesias, and Chvostek's or Trousseau's signs).[25]

Vitamin D deficiency, often due to insufficient sunlight exposure or inadequate dietary intake, is a common cause, impairing the absorption of calcium and phosphorus. The recommended daily intake of vitamin D is 400 International Units (IU). Malabsorption disorders, such as celiac disease, inflammatory bowel disease, and gastrointestinal bypass surgery, can also lead to osteomalacia by hindering nutrient absorption.[25–27] Additionally, hereditary conditions, such as hereditary hypophosphatemic rickets syndromes (eg, X-linked hypophosphatemic rickets) and renal disorders, such as renal tubular acidosis or chronic kidney disease, may contribute to development of osteomalacia.[28–30] Tumor-induced osteomalacia, a rare form of the disease, results from tumors producing excess fibroblast growth factor 23, disrupting phosphate and vitamin D metabolism.[31] Finally, chronic exposure to elevated levels of metal and minerals such as fluoride may result in fluorosis, a disorder of skeletal and dental health, through the direct inhibition of mineralization within bones and tooth enamel.[32] However, fluoride-induced osteomalacia is uncommon and associated with chronic exposure to very high levels of fluoride, often well beyond levels typically encountered in drinking water or dental products. Understanding and addressing the underlying cause is crucial for effective management and treatment of osteomalacia.

When osteomalacia occurs in childhood, it is accompanied by rickets, which is characterized by the widening of epiphyses, delayed growth, bowed legs, cranio-tabes, delayed fontanel closure, dental issues, and delayed motor development, in addition to the symptoms seen in adults.[33,34] It is important to differentiate rickets from other conditions that may present with similar features, such as skeletal dysplasia, liver disease, and primary hypoparathyroidism.[35] While the risk factors for development of osteomalacia are the same at any age, it is important to consider additional risk factors for rickets, such as exclusive breastfeeding without vitamin D supplementation (due to innately low levels present in breast milk), darker skin pigmentation (as less vitamin D is produced in response to sunlight exposure), and premature birth (due to lower vitamin storage).[36]

Evaluation

There is no single laboratory finding specific for osteomalacia. Patients with osteomalacia will typically exhibit hypophosphatemia or hypocalcemia. Increased alkaline phosphatase activity is also characteristic of diseases with impaired osteoid mineralization and may be of diagnostic value. Unfortunately, osteomalacia lacks distinctive lab and imaging criteria for diagnosis. Given clinical presentation is often non-specific, Uday and Hogler[37] proposed diagnostic criteria to include elevated parathyroid hormone levels, elevated alkaline phosphatase, low urine calcium, low calcium intake (<300 mg/day), and low calcidiol levels (<30 nmol/L). These criteria are specifically useful in the absence of liver or kidney disease. However, iliac crest bone biopsy is considered the criterion standard for diagnosis of osteomalacia. If a patient's bone pain persists despite appropriate treatment for presumed hypophosphatemic rickets and there is evidence of renal phosphate wasting, clinicians should consider further workup for more rare causes of osteomalacia. Primary forms of renal phosphate wasting include several genetic forms, tumor-induced osteomalacia, and Fanconi syndrome.

Management

Treatment of osteomalacia focuses on determining the etiology. For rickets prevention, 600 IU of vitamin D during pregnancy and 400 IU daily for infants after birth is recommended, in addition to monitoring in antenatal and child health surveillance programs.[37] High-risk populations require lifelong supplementation and food fortification with vitamin D or calcium.[37] Recommended treatment for adult patients with severe vitamin D deficiency (<12 ng/mL or 30 nmol/L) is 50,000 IU of oral ergocalciferol (vitamin D_2) or cholecalciferol (vitamin D_3) 1 day per week for 8 to 12 weeks, followed by 800 to 2000 IU of vitamin D_3 daily. Increases in urine calcium excretion and BMD are markers of healing from osteomalacia. Although serum calcium and phosphate may normalize after a few weeks, bone alkaline phosphatase may stay elevated for several months.[38]

Paget Disease

Background and prevalence

Paget disease of the bone, also known as osteitis deformans, is a rare chronic bone disorder characterized by abnormal and excessive remodeling of bone tissue. This disease is estimated to affect 1% to 2% of the US population.[39] This condition results in enlarged, weakened, and deformed bones. Paget disease can affect 1 or more bones in the body but most commonly involves the spine, pelvis, skull, and long bones.[40] In Paget disease, there is an abnormal increase in bone-resorbing cell (osteoclasts) activity, leading to excessive bone breakdown. The body responds by attempting to rebuild the bone, but the new bone is often structurally disorganized and weaker than healthy bone. This ongoing cycle of increased bone turnover results in enlarged and misshapen bones. Paget disease is often asymptomatic, and many individuals may not be aware of the condition. When symptoms do occur, they can include bone pain, joint pain, and deformities, such as enlargement of the skull, spinal stenosis, and bowing deformities of the long bones. Other symptoms may include warmth over affected bones, hearing loss (if the skull is involved), and neurologic symptoms (if there is compression of nearby nerves).[39,40]

Evaluation
Diagnosis is typically made through a combination of clinical evaluation, radiographic imaging studies (X-ray and dual-energy X-ray absorptiometry), and blood tests to measure alkaline phosphatase, which is often elevated in Paget disease. Many times, this disease is discovered incidentally on radiography with the presence of lytic lesions and sclerotic findings. Other hallmark signs include osteoporosis circumscripta in the skull, flame-shaped lesion in the long bones, osteolytic lesions near thickened lesions, bowed limbs, and fractures.[41]

Management
While treatment is not always necessary, medications to regulate bone turnover, such as bisphosphonates (first line) or calcitonin (second line for patients intolerant of bisphosphanates), may be used, along with pain management.[40] Regular monitoring, early detection, and appropriate intervention are essential aspects of managing Paget disease to prevent complications and optimize bone health. Patients with Paget disease often benefit from a multidisciplinary approach involving orthopedic specialists, endocrinologists, and other health care professionals.

Endocrine Disorders

Endocrine disturbances such as hyperparathyroidism, hyperthyroidism, and hypogonadism can also impact the skeletal system. Estrogen plays a primary role in bone formation and protection in both women and men, and deficiencies can lead to increased bone turnover and enhanced resorption, thereby resulting in osteoporosis.[42] Many postmenopausal women develop osteoporosis due to a decline in estrogen.[42] In adult

Table 2
Laboratory evaluation for suspected metabolic bone disease

Serum Studies	Urine Studies
Complete blood count	Urinalysis
Complete metabolic panel	24 h urine calcium
Calcium	24 h urine creatinine
Phosphate	
Alkaline phosphatase	
25-hydroxyvitamin D (calcidiol)	
Parathyroid hormone	
Testosterone	
Estradiol	
Transglutaminase immunoglobulin A antibody	
Thyroid-stimulating hormone	

men with acquired hypogonadism, estrogen deficiency may contribute more to bone loss than androgen deficiency, particularly if levels are below 10 to 15 pg/mL. Physicians should consider screening men aged 50 years and up hypogonadism, along with other risk factors are present; the threshold to screen men age 70 years and up is lower and may be appropriate with only one risk factor present. [43] Similarly, chronically elevated levels of parathyroid hormone seen in primary, secondary, and tertiary hyperparathyroidism stimulate the release of calcium from bone, resulting in decreased BMD.[44] The differential for secondary hyperparathyroidism remains broad as it may develop from a myriad of primary disorders, such as malignancy, chronic renal disease, malabsorption, and intestinal diseases (eg, celiac disease).[45] Clinicians should consider an underlying endocrine disorder if other evidence of MBD exists, and the primary disorder should be managed appropriately.

SUMMARY

Endocrine disorders such as hyperparathyroidism, hyperthyroidism, and hypogonadism negatively impact bone health. Health care professionals must be adept at identifying individuals at risk, conducting thorough evaluations, and crafting personalized treatment strategies. Disruptions in endocrine balance can lead to MBDs, characterized by a variety of skeletal issues and an increased risk of fractures. Vitamin D is crucial in regulating calcium and phosphate levels, facilitating their absorption, reabsorption, and mobilization in the body. Early identification of patients at elevated risk for bone diseases through screening is essential.

In managing osteoporosis, individuals with low BMD (T-score between −1.0 and −2.5) and high fracture risk, as assessed by FRAX, are recommended for treatment, aiming primarily to reduce fracture risks. Emerging therapies, such as romosozumab and odanacatib, are under investigation. Periodic monitoring of bone health, possibly every 4 years, is also suggested. Addressing osteomalacia effectively requires understanding and treating its specific causes. Risk factors include nutritional deficiencies, limited sun exposure, and certain birth conditions. Primary reasons for renal phosphate wasting include genetic issues, tumor-induced osteomalacia, and Fanconi syndrome. Recovery indicators such as calcium and phosphate levels may normalize quickly, but bone alkaline phosphatase levels could remain elevated longer. Symptoms can range from bone warmth to hearing loss and neurologic complications, depending on the affected area. For conditions like Paget disease, a multidisciplinary approach involving various specialists is advantageous. Clinicians should also explore underlying endocrine disorders when MBD symptoms are present, ensuring appropriate management of the primary condition. Routine biochemical tests to evaluate for underlying bone disease should include evaluation as illustrated in **Table 2**.

CLINICS CARE POINTS

- Dual X-ray absorptiometry (DEXA) screening is recommended for women aged 65 years or older, men aged 70 years or older, and postmenopausal women and men older than 50 years of age, depending on their risk factor profile.
- Treat osteoporosis in patients with low bone density (T-score between −1.0 and −2.5) who have a 3% or greater chance of hip fracture or 20% or greater chance of significant fracture (measured by FRAX) related to osteoporosis over the next 10 years.
- Testosterone treatment is advised for men with a high risk of osteoporotic fractures who exhibit testosterone levels below 200 ng/dL.

ACKNOWLEDGMENTS

The Scientific Publications staff at Mayo Clinic provided copyediting, proofreading, administrative, and clerical support.

DISCLOSURE

The authors have no conflicts of interest to disclose.

REFERENCES

1. Hart NH, Newton RU, Tan J, et al. Biological basis of bone strength: anatomy, physiology and measurement. J Musculoskelet Neuronal Interact 2020;20: 347–71.
2. Gilbert SF. Osteogenesis: the development of bones. In: Developmental biology. 6th ed. Sunderland, MA: Sinauer Associates; 2000.
3. Fleet JC. The role of vitamin D in the endocrinology controlling calcium homeostasis. Mol Cell Endocrinol 2017;453:36–45.
4. Sozen T, Ozisik L, Basaran NC. An overview and management of osteoporosis. Eur J Rheumatol 2017;4:46–56.
5. Kanis JA, Johnell O, Oden A, et al. Ten year probabilities of osteoporotic fractures according to BMD and diagnostic thresholds. Osteoporos Int 2001;12:989–95.
6. Sarafrazi N, Wambogo EA, Shepherd JA. Osteoporosis or low bone mass in older adults: United States, 2017–2018. NCHS data brief. No 405. Hyattsville, MD: National Center for Health Statistics, 2021. Available at: https://www.cdc.gov/nchs/data/databriefs/db405-H.pdf.
7. Kanis JA, Johansson H, Oden A, et al. A family history of fracture and fracture risk: a meta-analysis. Bone 2004;35:1029–37.
8. Buckley L, Guyatt G, Fink HA, et al. 2017 American college of rheumatology guideline for the prevention and treatment of glucocorticoid-induced osteoporosis. Arthritis Care Res (Hoboken) 2017;69:1095–110.
9. Shahinian VB, Kuo YF, Freeman JL, et al. Risk of fracture after androgen deprivation for prostate cancer. N Engl J Med 2005;352:154–64.
10. Klotzbuecher CM, Ross PD, Landsman PB, Abbott TA, Berger M. Patients with prior fractures have an increased risk of future fractures: a summary of the literature and statistical synthesis. J Bone Miner Res 2000;15:721–39.
11. Sullivan SD, Lehman A, Nathan NK, et al. Age of menopause and fracture risk in postmenopausal women randomized to calcium + vitamin D, hormone therapy, or the combination: results from the Women's Health Initiative Clinical Trials. Menopause 2017;24:371–8.
12. Cosman F, de Beur SJ, LeBoff MS, et al. Erratum to: Clinician's guide to prevention and treatment of osteoporosis. Osteoporos Int 2015;26:2045–7.
13. Cosman F, de Beur SJ, LeBoff MS, et al. Clinician's guide to prevention and treatment of osteoporosis. Osteoporos Int 2014;25:2359–81.
14. De Laet C, Kanis JA, Oden A, et al. Body mass index as a predictor of fracture risk: a meta-analysis. Osteoporos Int 2005;16:1330–8.
15. Watts NB, Adler RA, Bilezikian JP, et al. Osteoporosis in men: an endocrine society clinical practice guideline. J Clin Endocrinol Metab 2012;97:1802–22.
16. Unnanuntana A, Gladnick BP, Donnelly E, et al. The assessment of fracture risk. J Bone Joint Surg Am 2010;92:743–53.

17. FRAX Fracture Risk Assessment Tool. Centre for metabolic bone diseases, University of Sheffield. Available at: https://frax.shef.ac.uk/FRAX/tool.aspx? country=9. [Accessed 15 December 2023].
18. Tu KN, Lie JD, Wan CKV, et al. Osteoporosis: A Review of Treatment Options. P T 2018;43:92–104.
19. Bauer DC, Schwartz A, Palermo L, et al. Fracture prediction after discontinuation of 4 to 5 years of alendronate therapy: the FLEX study. JAMA Intern Med 2014; 174:1126–34.
20. Camacho PM, Petak SM, Binkley N, et al. American association of clinical endocrinologists and american college of endocrinology clinical practice guidelines for the diagnosis and treatment of postmenopausal osteoporosis - 2016. Endocr Pract 2016;22:1–42.
21. Trovas GP, Lyritis GP, Galanos A, et al. A randomized trial of nasal spray salmon calcitonin in men with idiopathic osteoporosis: effects on bone mineral density and bone markers. J Bone Miner Res 2002;17:521–7.
22. Management of osteoporosis in postmenopausal women: the 2021 position statement of The North American Menopause Society. Menopause 2021;28:973–97.
23. Berry SD, Samelson EJ, Pencina MJ, et al. Repeat bone mineral density screening and prediction of hip and major osteoporotic fracture. JAMA 2013; 310:1256–62.
24. Gourlay ML, Fine JP, Preisser JS, et al. Bone-density testing interval and transition to osteoporosis in older women. N Engl J Med 2012;366:225–33.
25. Cianferotti L. Osteomalacia is not a single disease. Int J Mol Sci 2022;23.
26. Frame B, Parfitt AM. Osteomalacia: current concepts. Ann Intern Med 1978;89: 966–82.
27. Karefylakis C, Naslund I, Edholm D, et al. Vitamin D status 10 years after primary gastric bypass: gravely high prevalence of hypovitaminosis D and raised PTH levels. Obes Surg 2014;24:343–8.
28. Alon U, Chan JC. Effects of hydrochlorothiazide and amiloride in renal hypophosphatemic rickets. Pediatrics 1985;75:754–63.
29. Econs MJ, McEnery PT. Autosomal dominant hypophosphatemic rickets/osteomalacia: clinical characterization of a novel renal phosphate-wasting disorder. J Clin Endocrinol Metab 1997;82:674–81.
30. Murthy AS. X-linked hypophosphatemic rickets and craniosynostosis. J Craniofac Surg 2009;20:439–42.
31. Seemann L, Padala SA, Mohammed A, et al. Tumor-induced osteomalacia and the importance of plasma fibroblast growth factor 23 as an indicator: diagnostic delay leads to a suicide attempt. J Investig Med High Impact Case Rep 2019;7. 2324709619895162.
32. Wang Y, Yin Y, Gilula LA, et al. Endemic fluorosis of the skeleton: radiographic features in 127 patients. AJR Am J Roentgenol 1994;162:93–8.
33. Francis RM, Selby PL. Osteomalacia. Baillieres Clin Endocrinol Metab 1997;11: 145–63.
34. Pitt MJ. Rickets and osteomalacia are still around. Radiol Clin North Am 1991;29: 97–118.
35. Mortier GR, Cohn DH, Cormier-Daire V, et al. Nosology and classification of genetic skeletal disorders: 2019 revision. Am J Med Genet 2019;179:2393–419.
36. Wagner CL, Greer FR, American Academy of Pediatrics Section on Breastfeeding, American Academy of Pediatrics Committee on Nutrition. Prevention of rickets and vitamin d deficiency in infants, children, and adolescents. Pediatrics 2008;122:1142–52.

37. Uday S, Hogler W. Spot the silent sufferers: A call for clinical diagnostic criteria for solar and nutritional osteomalacia. J Steroid Biochem Mol Biol 2019;188:141–6.
38. Allen SC, Raut S. Biochemical recovery time scales in elderly patients with osteomalacia. J R Soc Med 2004;97:527–30.
39. Tiegs RD. Paget disease of bone. In: NORD guide to rare disorders. Philadelphia, PA: Lippincott Williams & Wilkins; 2003. p. 24–5.
40. Ralston SH, Langston AL, Reid IR. Pathogenesis and management of Paget's disease of bone. Lancet 2008;372:155–63.
41. Rianon NJ, des Bordes JK. Paget disease of bone for primary care. Am Fam Physician 2020;102:224–8.
42. Cheng CH, Chen LR, Chen KH. Osteoporosis due to hormone imbalance: an overview of the effects of estrogen deficiency and glucocorticoid overuse on bone turnover. Int J Mol Sci 2022;23.
43. Finkelstein JS, Lee H, Leder BZ, et al. Gonadal steroid-dependent effects on bone turnover and bone mineral density in men. J Clin Invest 2016;126:1114–25.
44. Silva BC, Bilezikian JP. Parathyroid hormone: anabolic and catabolic actions on the skeleton. Curr Opin Pharmacol 2015;22:41–50.
45. Husby S, Murray JA, Katzka DA. AGA clinical practice update on diagnosis and monitoring of celiac disease-changing utility of serology and histologic measures: expert review. Gastroenterology 2019;156:885–9.

Male Reproductive Endocrine Disorders

Matthew McCoskey, MD*, Nicholas Vernon, DO

KEYWORDS

- Hypogonadism • Gynecomastia • Erectile dysfunction • Low testosterone
- Exogenous testosterone supplementation • Hypothalamic–pituitary–gonadal axis

KEY POINTS

- Hypogonadism is diagnosed with symptomatic low total serum testosterone levels.
- Treatment of hypogonadism begins with lifestyle modifications targeted at reversing factors altering the hypothalamic–pituitary–gonadal axis.
- Exogenous testosterone supplementation can adversely cause infertility, polycythemia, and obstructive sleep apnea; the risks on major adverse cardiovascular events or prostate cancer are less clear.
- Gynecomastia results from a high estrogen-to-androgen ratio.
- The most common cause of male infertility is hypogonadism.

INTRODUCTION

The endocrine system impacts male health and sexuality with its intricate regulation of testosterone production and function. Maintaining the delicate balance of hormones is crucial for a man's well-being and reproductive capability; any disruption, such as hypogonadism or sexual dysfunctions, can have profound consequences. Understanding this complexity is essential in diagnosing and managing conditions that impact male sexual and hormonal health that may affect both physical and psychological aspects of masculinity.

PRIMARY AND SECONDARY HYPOGONADISM
Clinical Features

Male hypogonadism results from testes failing to secrete normal levels of testosterone or produce adequate levels of sperm which can either be caused by a disorder of the testes (primary hypogonadism) or a disorder of the hypothalamic–pituitary axis (secondary hypogonadism). Given that testosterone has numerous roles at different stages of maturity, testosterone deficiencies manifest differently based upon the stage of life.[1]

Department of Family Medicine, Tidelands Health, 4320 Holmestown Road, Myrtle Beach, SC 29588, USA
* Corresponding author.
E-mail address: mmccoskey@tidelandshealth.org

Prim Care Clin Office Pract 51 (2024) 455–466
https://doi.org/10.1016/j.pop.2024.04.003   **primarycare.theclinics.com**

- During fetal life, testosterone and its metabolites (primarily dihydrotestosterone) stimulate the development of the fetal penis and scrotum, including the descent of the testis into the scrotum. Thus, testosterone deficiency in fetal life results in ambiguous genitalia, micropenis, or cryptorchidism.
- During puberty, testosterone stimulates the development of secondary sexual characteristics responsible for the "masculinization" of the adolescent boy. Stimulated changes include hair and sebum proliferation, increased red blood cell production, muscle and bone development including closure of epiphyseal plates, and vocal cord thickening resulting in lower pitched voice changes. Prepubertal testosterone deficiencies (usually resulting from Klinefelter syndrome, pituitary injury, or testicular insult such as radiation, infection, or toxic exposures) result in delayed or incomplete puberty changes including scant pubic hair, inability to grow a full beard, gynecomastia, osteoporosis, and infertility.
- In adulthood, testosterone maintains the masculine changes achieved in puberty. Age-related hypogonadism or so-called "late-onset hypogonadism" is associated with decreased sexual libido, erectile dysfunction, brain fog, reduction in muscle mass, and reduction in bone density.[2]

Evaluation and Diagnosis

For symptomatic patients, evaluation should begin with a thorough history and physical examination to drive potential laboratory workup considering the patient's risk factors. Physical signs of testosterone deficiency include gynecomastia, underdeveloped secondary sexual characteristics (such as beard, pubic and axillary hair growth). Factors that may alter the hypothalamic–pituitary–gonadal axis are listed in **Box 1**.

Next, establish if a total serum testosterone level is below normal range (<300 ng/dL).[3] The blood drawn should be obtained in the absence of any acute illness that could give

Box 1
Conditions that can alter the hypothalamic–pituitary–gonadal axis
Alcoholism
Chronic inflammation
Depression
Diabetes mellitus
Genetic disorders (Kallman, Klinefelter, and Prader–Willi syndromes)
High cortisol levels and stress disorders
Infections
Intracranial processes affecting the pituitary or hypothalamic region
Liver disease
Malnutrition
Medications (steroids, opioids, marijuana)
Obesity
Prolactin excess
Testicular injury or radiation
Thyroid disorders

a spurious value and drawn between 8:00 to 10:00 AM as natural testosterone levels peak in the early morning hours. If total serum testosterone is low, then repeat total testosterone level with a luteinizing hormone (LH) level to differentiate between primary and secondary hypogonadism. Consider additional testing for differentiation between primary and secondary hypogonadism, as listed in **Table 1**.

Treatment

The goal of testosterone therapy is both to restore total testosterone levels to a range of 450 to 600 ng/dL and relieve symptoms attributed to hypogonadism.[3] Treatment options include the following:

- Lifestyle modifications should be implemented as a *first-line* testosterone therapy particularly aimed at reversing risk factors altering the hypothalamic–pituitary–gonadal axis and interfering with the natural production of testosterone.
  - *Achieve a healthy* body mass index (BMI): Adipose tissues produce estrogens which negatively feedback into the hypothalamic–pituitary–gonadal axis suppressing gonadotropins.[4] Substantial weight loss can result in increased levels of gonadotropins and testosterone in obesity-related hypogonadism; however, excessively restrictive diets are less effective at reversing androgen deficiencies.[5]
  - *Participate in regular cardio and strength training exercises*: Moderate physical exercise results in increased testosterone levels[6]; though high-intensity endurance training with caloric deprivation causes suppression of gonadotropins.[1]
  - *Manage comorbidities*: Chronic diseases are associated with low testosterone. The metabolic derangements of organ failure especially from liver disease, chronic kidney disease, diabetes, congestive heart failure, and chronic lung disease can impact testosterone levels.[1]
  - *Improved sleep hygiene*: Total sleep deprivation is associated with lower testosterone levels.[7]

Table 1
Secondary testing for hypogonadism

Condition	Total Serum Testosterone Level	Luteinizing Hormone Level	Additional Testing to Consider
Primary hypogonadism	<300 ng/dL	Above normal	• Karyotype to rule out Klinefelter syndrome
Secondary hypogonadism	<300 ng/dL	Normal or reduced	• Prolactin level to evaluate for hyperprolactinemia • Estradiol level (especially in patients with gynecomastia) as a high estrogen state can suppress LH, thus secondarily lowering testosterone production. • Morning cortisol level (drawn between 7:00AM to 9:00AM); high cortisol levels inhibit testosterone • Serum ferritin and transferrin levels to rule out hemochromatosis • MRI of sella if concern for pituitary mass

○ *Managing stress*: Chronic stress inhibits testosterone production and spermatogenesis.[8]
○ *Eat a nutritious diet rich in phytonutrients*: Various micronutrient deficiencies can impact testosterone synthesis including boron, magnesium, vitamin D, and zinc.[9] Dietary fat is essential for testosterone production and recommended daily allowances are above 25% of macronutrients.[9]
- Exogenous testosterone supplementation is a *second-line* therapy.
○ Multiple testosterone formulations are available with different delivery methods and variable pricing.
  ■ *Transdermal gels and solutions* rubbed into the skin on shoulders, arms, thighs, or axilla avoids the use of needles, but some individuals incompletely absorb the testosterone. Also, physical contact may inadvertently transfer the gel or solution to others including young children or women.
  ■ *Injectable testosterone* is available in long- and short-acting forms. Lower doses given at shorter intervals can create a more physiologic testosterone serum level, though it would require the patient to inject themselves more frequently. Conversely, larger spaced-out doses give fewer injections but more variability in peaks and nadirs. Some preparations with oil vehicles carry black box warnings for serious pulmonary oil microembolism reactions.
  ■ *Implanted testosterone pellets* that are injected by clinicians into the buttock or flank offers a longer interval between dosing (usually 3–4 months) but requires a minor in-office procedure with specialty equipment and training.
  ■ Currently, no oral options are approved by the US Food and Drug Administration (FDA) except a mucosally absorbed *buccal patch* applied to upper gums twice a day. A common adverse effect is mouth irritation.
  ■ *Nasal spray* dose 3 times a day can cause some nasal irritation and rhinorrhea.
○ For patients on exogenous testosterone supplementation, initial follow-up should be based on clinician preference but further recommendations to monitor total testosterone levels are set at every 6 to 12 months to titrate dosing. The target total serum testosterone range is 450 to 600 ng/dL and one should recognize that supplementation feeds back into the hypothalamic–pituitary–gonadal axis suppressing endogenous production of testosterone and spermatogenesis. Reproductive age men should be advised that exogenous testosterone supplementation carries a significant infertility risk which may be long lasting. A reproductive health evaluation is recommended for reproductive age men with testosterone deficiency prior to exogenous testosterone supplementation.[3]
○ Exogenous testosterone supplementation increases the risk for polycythemia; thus, clinicians should check hemoglobin and hematocrit levels prior to initiating supplementation and monitor levels periodically to assess for excessive erythrocytosis.[3,10]
○ Further research is needed to advise on exogenous testosterone supplementation's effect on major adverse cardiovascular events such as myocardial infarction, stroke, and cardiovascular mortality. Current scientific literature is inconsistent as multiple studies including randomized control trials disagree about the link between testosterone therapy and possible increased cardiovascular risk.[2,3] Confoundingly, untreated low testosterone levels are associated with an increased risk of cardiovascular events which some argue is because both are secondary to poor overall health. Currently, package inserts

for testosterone products warn that they may increase the risk of major adverse cardiovascular events. It is unclear whether this is a class effect or whether different delivery methods are less safe. For example, Allergan has discontinued manufacturing Androderm transdermal patches after a settlement in 2018 where plaintiffs claimed serious side effects from the transdermal patches including cardiac death.[11]

- o Additionally, further research is needed to advise on exogenous testosterone supplementation's effect on the development of prostate cancer as the link between the two is controversial. The American Urologic Association recommends checking prostate specific antigen (PSA) prior to initiating supplementation in those over the age of 40 years. Screen for lower urinary tract symptoms secondary to prostate enlargement at follow-up visits.[3]
- o Exogenous testosterone supplementation may induce or worsen obstructive sleep apnea; consider evaluating a sleep study when indicated.[1]
- *Third-line* alternative or augmenting therapies include
  - o Human chorionic gonadotropin (hCG) injections are active on the same receptors as LH which stimulates Leydig cells to produce testosterone.[1] This treatment requires psychologically normally functioning testis. Chorionic gonadotropin injections hold FDA approval for use in male patients with hypogonadotropic hypogonadism and pediatric patients with cryptorchidism.[3]
  - o Although not FDA-approved in male patients, selective estrogen receptor modulators (SERM; such as clomiphene citrate or tamoxifen) inhibit the negative feedback of estradiol on LH production thus resulting in greater stimulation of Leydig cells to produce testosterone and are used off-label for spermatogenesis induction.[3]
  - o Although not FDA-approved in male patients, aromatase inhibitors (such as anastrozole) block the conversion of testosterone to estradiol. Avoid prolonged use given concern for inducing osteoporosis.[3]

GYNECOMASTIA
Clinical Features

Gynecomastia is the benign enlargement of glandular tissue of the male breast, not to be confused with pseudogynecomastia which is breast enlargement from the increase of adipose tissues without glandular enlargement.[1] On palpation, glandular tissue feels rubbery, loosely anchored, lobular, and located deep to the nipple and areola. Conversely, pseudogynecomastia is softer, with coarser lobular architecture that is loose and relatively more dispersed subcutaneously. An alternative differential of male breast enlargement is breast cancer, which is more commonly unilateral, asymmetrical, hard with tethered skin changes, or nipple discharge.

Evaluation and Diagnosis

Gynecomastia results from a high estrogen-to-androgen ratio which can be secondary to either a high estrogen level or low androgen levels or rarely both.[12] Estrogen and progesterone hormones stimulate the growth and development of breast glandular tissues, while androgens inhibit their growth. Transient gynecomastia is relatively common in the neonatal period when excess maternal estrogens remain in baby boys or in early pubertal boys when excess estrogen production outpaces the onset of increased testosterone production.

Gynecomastia is generally diagnosed solely on a physical examination.[1] Pathologic gynecomastia that is either larger than 5 cm, rapidly expanding, or symptomatic should be worked up to identify the cause of estrogen excess or androgen deficiency. Evaluation begins with a history and physical examination with emphasis on potential predisposing conditions or medications (**Table 2**).

Initial laboratory evaluation usually involves serum testosterone level, estradiol, LH, hCG, and thyroid-stimulating hormone (TSH). Consider checking follicle-stimulating hormone (FSH), prolactin, and/or karyotyping if indicated.

Imaging is usually not indicated unless malignancy is suspected as evidenced by suspicious palpable breast mass, axillary adenopathy, nipple discharge, or nipple retraction or for an indeterminate palpable breast mass.[13] The preferred method of imaging is either diagnostic mammography or ultrasound.

Treatment

Transient gynecomastia in infancy is common and generally resolves in the first year of life without treatment or workup.[14] Half of prepubescent boys will have some degree of gynecomastia; roughly 90% of those patients will have complete resolution within 24 to 48 months without treatment.[14]

For gynecomastia in adolescents or adults, treatment is based upon underlying cause, noting that long-standing gynecomastia may result in progressive stromal fibrosis that is only rarely reversed with conservative interventions. Breast reduction surgery can be considered if there are significant physical symptoms or emotional distress despite removal of offending reason(s) for estrogen excess or androgen deficiency. SERM, aromatase inhibitors, and androgen are all options in the treatment of gynecomastia depending on the causative factors though each possess significant risk of adverse effects.[15]

Pseudogynecomastia is best treated with weight loss, and if necessary, liposuction to decrease adipose deposits overlying the pectoralis muscles.[16]

ENDOCRINE CAUSES OF SEXUAL DYSFUNCTION
Clinical Features

Hormones regulate sexual development and function. Excluding psychological problems (such as depression, relationship tensions, intimacy issues), endocrine dysregulations are a primary source for sexual dysfunction.

- *Libido disorders* are persistently low sexual desire causing significant distress in the patient or their partner. Often libidinal problems are multifactorial and comorbid with psychological disorders.
  - Androgen deficiency: Low serum testosterone is associated with hypoactive sexual libido.

Table 2	
Underlying causes for gynecomastia	
Causes of Estrogen Excess	**Causes of Androgen Deficiency**
• Exposure to exogenous estrogen • Estrogen receptor agonists (marijuana, digitoxin, phthalates) • Aromatase excess • Endocrine tumors (secreting estrogen or hCG) • Cirrhosis	• Primary or secondary hypogonadism • Elevated prolactin (prolactinoma, medication effect such as from antipsychotics, sedatives, antidepressants) • Drugs altering androgen action (spironolactone, 5a-reductase inhibitors, H2 blockers) • Androgen resistance

- ○ Hyperprolactinemia results in loss of libido; likely secondary to inhibition of testosterone production.[17]
- ○ Thyroid disorders: Hypothyroidism can cause sexual dysfunction in the form of delayed orgasm, erectile dysfunction or poor-quality erections, and poor energy level thus reducing stamina and libido. Hypothyroidism can also predispose a patient to weight gain, which can have a compounding effect on sexual dysfunction. Hyperthyroidism, the other end of the spectrum, can cause premature ejaculation.[18]
- ○ Metabolic syndrome is characterized by increased waist circumference, hypertension, hypertriglyceridemia, low high-density lipoprotein, and resistance to insulin. Metabolic syndrome is associated with hypogonadism, increased fatigue, and diminished sexual desire.[19]
- ○ Certain medications can adversely affect libido especially opioids and antidepressants. Narcotic-induced androgen insufficiency occurs when opioids inhibit the hypothalamus–pituitary axis, leading to reduced levels of gonadotropins.[20] Selective serotonin reuptake inhibitors may cause sexual dysfunction in 40% to 65% of patients, especially paroxetine users.[21]
- *Erectile dysfunction* is defined as the difficulty attaining or maintaining sufficient penile rigidity interfering with sexual performance. Erectile dysfunction is often a harbinger for subclinical cardiovascular disease, and men with erectile dysfunction are 1.3 to 1.6 times more likely to have a cardiovascular event in the next 10 years compared to men without erectile dysfunction and these cardiovascular events are more likely to be fatal.[1,22] Diabetes mellitus can result in dysregulated autonomics, endothelial degradation, neuropathies, and alterations in energy levels. These all can have profound effects on the ability to engage in sex.[22] Erectile dysfunction and hypogonadism are often comorbid together, and although exogenous testosterone supplementation is not an effective monotherapy for erectile dysfunction, it has been observed that in patients with total testosterone less than 300 ng/dL and erectile dysfunction that exogenous testosterone supplementation combined with phosphodiesterase inhibitor is more effective than phosphodiesterase inhibitor treatment alone.[22]
- *Ejaculatory disorders (premature, delayed, or anejaculation)*: Mechanically, ejaculation is regulated by various neurotransmitters; 5HT serotonin delays ejaculation while dopamine and oxytocin stimulate it. The serotonin hypothesis theorizes that changes in receptor sensitivities manipulate thresholds. Selective serotonin reuptake inhibitors and steroid 5a-reductase inhibitors can prolong intravaginal ejaculatory latencies.[1]

Evaluation and Diagnosis

The workup for sexual dysfunctions focuses on a detailed medical, sexual, and psychosocial history, and physical examination to rule out nonendocrine causes (including psychiatric illnesses as these may be more important to address first) followed by targeted laboratory investigations if warranted.

- If signs of hypogonadism, check morning total testosterone level with reflex to LH if testosterone level is low.
- Hyperprolactinemia is rare, so checking prolactin levels is low yield unless the patient has a low total testosterone level.[17]
- Consider checking TSH with reflex to Triiodothyronine (T3) and Thyroxine (T4) if thyroid dysfunction is suspected.

- Consider metabolic workup including glucose or hemoglobin A1c (A1c) to exclude diabetes if suspected.

Treatment

Treatment is based upon the underlying root cause.

- If comorbid psychological disorders, consider referral to a mental health professional for whole person care.
- For patients with erectile dysfunction associated with metabolic syndrome, clinicians should educate patients on lifestyle modifications that can improve overall health and thus impact erectile function.[22] Healthy lifestyle choices include exercising regularly, eating well-balanced meals, limiting meat consumption, limiting alcohol, and avoiding smoking.
- Oral phosphodiesterase type 5 inhibitors (sildenafil, tadalafil, vardenafil, and avanafil) are FDA-approved for erectile dysfunction. Avoid concurrent nitrates. Sildenafil and vardenafil are less effective after large meals. For men who fail a trial of phosphodiesterase type 5 inhibitors, consider a referral to urology for alternative second-line treatments such as vacuum erection devices, intraurethral alprostadil, intracavernosal injections, or penile prosthesis implants.[23]

ENDOCRINE CAUSES OF INFERTILITY
Clinical Features

Infertility is the failure to achieve a pregnancy after 12 months or more of regular unprotected sexual intercourse. Male infertility, estimated to affect approximately 7% of men, results from decreased levels of sperm production, abnormal sperm morphology and motility, or problems with ejaculation.[1,23]

- The most common cause of male infertility is hypogonadism. LH, FSH, and testosterone are all required to induce Sertoli cell proliferation, grow and maintain the testis, and stimulate spermatogenesis.[24] Dysregulations in the hypothalamic–pituitary–gonadal axis interfere with sperm production. Exogenous testosterone (whether prescribed or the illicit use of anabolic steroids for bodybuilding) suppresses endogenous gonadotropin resulting in oligozoospermia or azoospermia.
- Ionizing radiation, chemotherapy, and environmental exposures that damage Sertoli cells (including bisphenol A [BPA], dioxin, dichlorodiphenyltrichloroethane [DDT], phthalates, certain fungicides) impact sperm count and morphology.[25]
- Disorders that obstruct the reproductive tract blocking the path of semen (such as congenital bilateral absence of vas deferens, cystic fibrosis, postinfectious fibrosis of vas deferens) interfere with sperm transport.[1]

Evaluation and Diagnosis

Clinical evaluation should focus on risk factors for male infertility including evidence of androgen deficiency, medications that may interfere with hypothalamic–pituitary–gonadal axis, and sexual history especially any genitourinary infections. Examine the scrotum and testes for varicocele, mass, or vas deferens pathology. Laboratory testing is centered on serum total testosterone, LH, FSH levels and semen analysis with sperm count, morphology, and motility.

Treatment

- For primary hypogonadism, fertility treatment options are limited as hormonal treatments are usually ineffective. Consider referring to a fertility specialist for evaluation and possible assisted reproductive treatments such as in vitro fertilization or intrauterine insemination.[1]

- For secondary hypogonadism, if possible, remove stimulus suppressing gonadotropins and consider stimulating sperm production with gonadotropin or GnRH treatments.[26]
- For some disorders of sperm transport, sperm can be retrieved from ejaculate or aspirated from epididymis for implantation via assisted reproductive treatments.

TRANSGENDER ENDOCRINOLOGY
Discussion

Individuals whose gender identification does not match their physical sexual characteristics may seek endocrine therapy for gender transition via suppression of endogenous hormones and/or addition of exogenous agents. The general goal of treatment is to reduce gender dysphoria and psychological stress associated with it; however, these treatments are not benign in nature and significant forethought must be given prior to treatment especially as many effects may be permanent or only partially reversible.

Transgender Health Disparities

Gender dysphoria is associated with numerous mental health comorbidities. Compared to cisgender peers, patients who identify as transgender are at higher risk for.

- Anxiety, depression, or affective disorders
- Self-injuries and suicide attempts
- Use of drugs or alcohol
- Homelessness
- Sexually transmitted infections[27–29]

Gender-affirming Hormone Therapy

- General considerations
  - Consider tertiary care referral for multispecialty services prior to and during treatment to include endocrinology, psychiatry, and mental health counselors.
  - Not all states and localities legally allow medical or surgical treatment for gender transition, especially for minors. Check with your state or locality's laws regarding age restrictions and requirements prior to starting therapy.[28]
  - Patients with a history of deep vein thrombosis or pulmonary embolism should have a hematologic workup prior to starting hormonal therapy.[30]
  - Pubertal blockers with gonadotropin hormone-releasing hormone (GnRH) agonists may adversely affect bone mineral density and fertility.[1]
- Male to female feminization treatments
  - Treatment usually involves exogenous estrogen supplementation plus an androgen antagonist (such as spironolactone, GnRH agonist, or cyproterone acetate).[28]
  - 17b-estradiol (vs conjugated or synthetic estrogens) is the preferred estrogen for ease of monitoring serum levels to titrate dosing. Also, synthetic estrogens carry an increased risk for venous thromboembolisms.[1]
  - The effect of increased serum estrogen levels results in breast tissue growth, fat redistribution around the hips, and decreased testicular volume.
  - Testosterone reduction results in decreased libido, decreased muscle mass, and an increase in erectile dysfunction.

- Downregulated FSH levels impact fertility through decreased spermatogenesis. Transgender women should be counseled on the option of preserving fertility via sperm cryopreservation before initiating treatment.[1]
- Exogenous estrogen significantly increases the risk of cerebral vascular accidents and venous thromboembolisms.[30]
- *Female to male* masculinization treatments
- Treatment usually involves exogenous testosterone supplementation.[28]
- The effect of increased serum testosterone levels results in permanent voice changes, increased body hair growth, male pattern hair thinning on the scalp, clitoromegaly, and increased libido.
- Estrogen suppression causes vaginal atrophy and dryness which can lead to chronic irritation and pain with vaginal intercourse.
- Usually, menstruation ceases on exogenous testosterone supplementation; however, infertility is not automatic and birth control should be considered especially as increased testosterone levels can adversely affect the fetus.
- Exogenous testosterone supplementation increases the risk for polycythemia, and hemoglobin levels should be monitored regularly as discussed elsewhere.[1]

CLINICS CARE POINTS

- Hypogonadism is diagnosed with a total serum testosterone level on multiple occasions less than 300 ng/dL along with symptoms.
- First-line treatment of hypogonadism involves lifestyle modifications targeted at reversing risk factors altering the hypothalamic–pituitary–gonadal axis.
- Exogenous testosterone supplementation carries a significant infertility risk as downregulated follicle-stimulating hormone levels decrease spermatogenesis.
- Gynecomastia results from a high estrogen-to-androgen ratio. In infancy and prepubescent boys, gynecomastia is predominantly transient. For gynecomastia in adolescents or adults, treatment is based upon underlying cause of estrogen excess or androgen deficiency.
- Erectile dysfunction is often a harbinger for subclinical cardiovascular disease.
- Exogenous testosterone supplementation is not an effective monotherapy for erectile dysfunction. If hypogonadism is comorbid, then testosterone with a phosphodiesterase inhibitor is more effective than phosphodiesterase inhibitor treatment alone.
- Infertility associated with primary hypogonadism rarely responds to hormonal treatments; rather consider referring to a fertility specialist for evaluation and possible assisted reproductive treatments.
- Hormone therapies for gender transition are not benign in nature and significant forethought must be given prior to treatment given its risks, permanence, and possible comorbid mental health issues. Treatment is best accomplished in a multidisciplinary setting.

DISCLOSURE

The authors have nothing to disclose.

REFERENCES

1. Bhasin S. and Basson R. Sexual Dysfunction in Men and Women, In: Melmed S, Auchus RJ, Goldfine AB, et al. Williams Textbook of Endocrinology, 14th edition, Elsevier - Health Sciences Division; Philadelphia, PA, 756–805.

2. Nguyen CP, Hirsch, Moeny, et al. Testosterone and "Age-Related Hypogonadism"–FDA Concerns. N Engl J Med 2015;373(8):689–91.
3. Mulhall JP, Trost LW, Brannigan RE, et al. Evaluation and management of testosterone deficiency: AUA guideline. J Urol 2018;200:423–32.
4. Hetemäki N, Mikkola, Tikkanen, et al. Adipose tissue estrogen production and metabolism in premenopausal women. J Steroid Biochem Mol Biol 2021;209: 105849.
5. Glass AR, Swerdloff RS, Bray GA, et al. Low serum testosterone and sex-hormone-binding-globulin in massively obese men. J Clin Endocrinol Metab 1977;45(6):1211–9.
6. Kumagai H, Zempo-Miyaki, Yoshikawa, et al. Increased physical activity has a greater effect than reduced energy intake on lifestyle modification-induced increases in testosterone. J Clin Biochem Nutr 2016;58(1):84–9.
7. Liang S, Si-Zheng Z, Jian Z, et al. Effect of partial and total sleep deprivation on serum testosterone in healthy males: a systematic review and meta-analysis. Sleep Med 2021;88:267–73.
8. Nargund VH. Effects of psychological stress on male fertility. Nat Rev Urol 2015; 12(7):373–82.
9. Zamir A, Ben-Zeev T, Hoffman JR. Manipulation of Dietary Intake on Changes in Circulating Testosterone Concentrations. Nutrients 2021 Sep 25;13(10):3375.
10. Petering RC, Brooks NA. Testosterone Therapy: Review of Clinical Applications. Am Fam Physician 2017 Oct 1;96(7):441–9.
11. Jensen L, "Testosterone Transdermal System" AHFS Clinical Drug Information 2023, Drug Information Service, University of Utah, Salt Lake City, UT. Available at Drug Shortage Detail: Testosterone Transdermal System (ashp.org). Accessed December 2, 2023.
12. Anawalt BD, Matsumoto AM. Aging and androgens: Physiology and clinical implications. Rev Endocr Metab Disord 2022;23(6):1123–37.
13. Niell BL, Niell, Lourenco, et al. ACR Appropriateness Criteria® Evaluation of the Symptomatic Male Breast. J Am Coll Radiol 2018;15:S313–9. Available at: https://acsearch.acr.org/docs/3091547/Narrative/. [Accessed 2 December 2023].
14. Kanakis GA, Nordkap L, Bang AK, et al. EAA clinical practice guidelines-gynecomastia evaluation and management. Andrology 2019;7(6):778–93.
15. Lapid O, van Wingerden JJ, Perlemuter L. Tamoxifen therapy for the management of pubertal gynecomastia: a systematic review. J Pediatr Endocrinol Metab 2013;26(9–10):803–7.
16. Dickson G. Gynecomastia. Am Fam Physician 2012;85(7):716–22.
17. Zeitlin SI, Rajfer J. Hyperprolactinemia and erectile dysfunction. Rev Urol 2000; 2(1):39–42.
18. Meikle AW. The interrelationships between thyroid dysfunction and hypogonadism in men and boys. Thyroid 2004;14 Suppl 1(Suppl 1):S17–25.
19. Tsujimura A. The Relationship between Testosterone Deficiency and Men's Health. World J Mens Health 2013;31(2):126–35.
20. Marudhai S, Patel M, Valaiyaduppu Subas S, et al. Long-term Opioids Linked to Hypogonadism and the Role of Testosterone Supplementation Therapy. Cureus 2020;12(10):e10813.
21. Jing E, Straw-Wilson K. Sexual dysfunction in selective serotonin reuptake inhibitors (SSRIs) and potential solutions: A narrative literature review. Ment Health Clin 2016;6(4):191–6.

22. Burnett AL, Nehra A, Breau RH, et al. Erectile dysfunction: AUA guideline. J Urol 2018;200:633–41.

23. Lindsay TJ, Vitrikas KR. Evaluation and Treatment of Infertility. Am Fam Physician 2015;91(5):308–14.

24. Shah W, Khan R, Shah B, et al. The Molecular Mechanism of Sex Hormones on Sertoli Cell Development and Proliferation. Front Endocrinol 2021;12:648141.

25. Gore AC, Chappell VA, Fenton SE, et al. Executive Summary to EDC-2: The Endocrine Society's Second Scientific Statement on Endocrine-Disrupting Chemicals. Endocr Rev 2015;36(6):593–602.

26. Ho CC, Tan HM. Treatment of the Hypogonadal Infertile Male-A Review. Sex Med Rev 2013;1(1):42–9.

27. Keo-Meier CL, Herman, Reisner, et al. Testosterone treatment and MMPI-2 improvement in transgender men: a prospective controlled study. J Consult Clin Psychol 2015;83(1):143–56.

28. Kerrebrouck M, Vantilborgh A, Collet S, et al. Thrombophilia and hormonal therapy in transgender persons: A literature review and case series. Int J Transgend Health 2022;23(4):377–91.

29. Coleman Eli, Bockting, Botzer, et al. Standards of Care for the Health of Transsexual, Transgender, and Gender-Nonconforming People, Version 7. Int J Transgenderism 2012;13(4):165–232.

30. Grant JM, Mottet LA, Tanis J, et al. Transgender discrimination survey.

Pituitary Disorders

Mark Owolabi, MD[a,*], Michael Malone, MD[b],
Andrew Merritt, MD[b]

KEYWORDS

- Pituitary • Cushing • Acromegaly • Insipidus • Oxytocin • Growth hormone
- Hyperthyroidism • Hypothyroidism

KEY POINTS

- Transsphenoidal sinus surgery is the first-line surgical therapy for most pituitary adenomas.
- Slow correction of hyponatremia in the setting of syndrome of inappropriate antidiuretic hormone release is essential as acute overcorrection can lead to severe central nervous system complications.
- The primary medical therapy for central diabetes insipidus is desmopressin.
- To avoid precipitating an adrenal crisis, all patients with central hypothyroidism should be evaluated and treated for adrenal insufficiency prior to initiating levothyroxine therapy.
- The treatment of choice for nearly all patients with hyperprolactinemic disorders is dopamine agonist therapy.

HYPOPITUITARISM

Hypopituitarism is a term for reduced pituitary gland function with varied causes including a pituitary tumor, head/brain injuries, head irradiation, stroke, medications, genetics, central nervous system (CNS) infections, inflammatory conditions, vasculitis, and Sheehan syndrome. Even with vague or nonspecific symptoms, there should be a low threshold for the evaluation of potential hypopituitarism in patients with these risk factors. We will briefly review Sheehan syndrome and empty sella syndrome, as these conditions can lead to variable deficiencies of pituitary hormones including pan-hypopituitarism.

Sheehan Syndrome

Introduction
Sheehan syndrome is a rare condition from postpartum ischemic anterior pituitary gland injury due to blood loss, hypovolemia, and shock.[1] Growth hormone (GH) is the most

[a] Department of Family Medicine, Medstar Health/Georgetown-Washington Hospital Center, 4151 Bladensburg Road, Colmar Manor, MD 20722, USA; [b] Department of Family Medicine, Tidelands Health Family Medicine Residency Program, 4320 Holmestown Road, Myrtle Beach, SC 29588, USA
* Corresponding author.
E-mail address: Mark.Owolabi9@gmail.com

common hormones affected by selective pituitary hypofunction, but panhypopituitarism is far more common in Sheehan syndrome. The hormones of the anterior pituitary are affected in a relatively predictable order when necrosis occurs. GH is impacted first and is followed by prolactin, follicle-stimulating hormone (FSH), luteinizing hormone (LH), adrenocorticotropic hormone (ACTH), and finally thyroid-stimulating hormone (TSH).[1] Although the posterior pituitary is rarely impacted, diabetes insipidus (DI) from reduced antidiuretic hormone (ADH) secretion has been infrequently reported.

Symptoms
The signs and symptoms of Sheehan syndrome can present hours to months after delivery with agalactorrhea being the first and most common symptom.[1] Other symptoms include amenorrhea or oligomenorrhea, hot flashes, decreased sex drive, fatigue, bradycardia, hypotension, cold intolerance, weight gain, weight loss, constipation, and loss of axillary and pubic hair.[1] The acute form can be dangerous if not recognized and treated quickly after childbirth. The persistent hypotension and tachycardia of adrenal dysfunction in Sheehan syndrome can mimic and be confused with hypovolemia and shock. However, hyponatremia and persistent hypoglycemia can help differentiate the diagnosis of Sheehan syndrome.[1]

Evaluation/diagnosis
Initial evaluation of anterior pituitary function is performed by obtaining bloodwork that includes a complete blood count, basic metabolic profile, TSH, FSH, LH, prolactin, estrogen, cortisol, and GH.[2] Diagnosis is based on low basal pituitary hormone level(s) along with a history and physical suggestive of Sheehan syndrome. Other laboratory abnormalities that may occur include anemia, thrombocytopenia, pancytopenia, hyponatremia, and hypoglycemia. An MRI evaluation of the pituitary should be performed to confirm the diagnosis.[3]

Treatment
The damage to the pituitary from Sheehan syndrome is usually permanent and pituitary hormone replacement therapy is typically lifelong. Referral to an endocrinologist who is familiar with hypopituitarism and Sheehan syndrome treatment is recommended.[4]

Complications
Possible severe complications include adrenal crisis and death.

Empty Sella Syndrome

Empty sella is a radiologic finding in which cerebral spinal fluid within the subarachnoid space compresses the pituitary gland in the sella turcica, making the space appear "empty."[5] When the finding of an empty sella is associated with low pituitary hormone levels, the condition is called empty sella syndrome.[5] The symptoms and treatment depend on the pituitary hormone deficiencies present.

SPECIFIC PITUITARY HORMONE DEFICIENCIES
Adrenocorticotropic Hormone

Adrenocorticotropic hormone (ACTH) is produced by the anterior pituitary in response to corticotropin-releasing hormone (CRH) released from the hypothalamus. CRH stimulates the release of ACTH, which acts on the adrenal cortex to regulate cortisol and androgen production.[6] Diseases associated with ACTH disorder of the pituitary include Cushing's syndrome (CS)/Cushing's disease (CD) and central adrenal insufficiency (CAI).[7] Pituitary insufficiency of ACTH production is usually the result of an adenoma that destroys the gland. It can also be caused by other conditions such as pituitary apoplexy or Sheehan syndrome.[8]

Adrenocorticotropic hormone deficiency: central adrenal insufficiency

CAI can be a life-threatening condition resulting in low cortisol levels and is caused by either pituitary disease or impaired hypothalamic function with inadequate CRH production. In this article, we will focus on CAI related to pituitary disease. ACTH deficiency with CAI may be isolated or, more frequently, occur in conjunction with other pituitary hormone deficiencies.[8]

Symptoms of central adrenal insufficiency. The signs and symptoms of CAI vary considerably and may include hypoglycemia, fatigue, lethargy, weakness, apnea, myalgias, weight loss, prolonged cholestatic jaundice, jitteriness, seizures, hypotension, vomiting, and hyponatremia without hyperkalemia. Hyperkalemia is only seen in primary adrenal insufficiency (PAI), as the renin–angiotensin–aldosterone system is intact.[8,9]

Evaluation/diagnosis. It is important to properly differentiate between CAI and PAI. CAI will only have low cortisol and sex steroids, but PAI will have deficiencies of cortisol, sex steroids, and aldosterone.

The diagnosis of CAI can be challenging. The initial evaluation of CAI is the measurement of a morning serum cortisol level and ACTH level. An elevated ACTH level with low cortisol indicates PAI, whereas a low or inappropriately normal ACTH value with low cortisol indicates CAI. dehydroepiandrosterone sulfate (DHEAS) testing may be helpful when AM cortisol and ACTH results are equivocal. A normal or high DHEAS level makes adrenal insufficiency unlikely.[10]

Unfortunately, these initial tests often cannot definitively establish the presence of adrenal insufficiency. In these cases, further testing with different stimulating agents and endocrinology consultation is needed.[8–10] The ACTH stimulation test is the best test to diagnose or exclude adrenal insufficiency and should be performed when baseline cortisol values are indeterminate.[9] Once diagnosis of CAI is made, a contrast-enhanced brain MRI is useful to detect pituitary masses and infectious or lymphocytic CNS disease.[10] Patients with CAI should also be evaluated for deficiencies or excess of other pituitary hormones.[9]

Treatment and complications. All individuals with CAI require glucocorticoid replacement therapy, which should be initiated and monitored in consultation with an endocrinologist.[9] Adrenal crisis is a life-threatening emergency that requires immediate treatment and should be suspected in patients who present with vasodilatory shock. Early recognition and correct management are mandatory to avoid significant morbidity and mortality and should not be delayed for diagnostic testing.[11]

Acute adrenal crisis is treated with intravenous (IV) glucocorticoid therapy and fluid resuscitation to correct hypovolemia and hyponatremia.[11] Dextrose-containing fluids can be used to improve hypoglycemia. If hypotension and hyponatremia is refractory to parenteral hydrocortisone and fluid administration, conditions other than adrenal crisis are the likely etiology.[11] Once the patient has stabilized, the steroid can be tapered over several days and converted to a maintenance regimen. The precipitating cause of adrenal crisis should be identified and treated appropriately.[11]

Adrenocorticotropic hormone excess: Cushing's disease

Background. CS is a rare disease due to persistently elevated plasma cortisol levels.[12] CD, is the most common cause of endogenous CS and is almost always caused by an ACTH-secreting pituitary tumor.[12]

Clinical manifestations. Common signs attributed to CD include weight gain in the face, midsection, and upper back. Other common features include facial plethora, muscle weakness, purple striae, easy bruising, immunosuppression, and osteopenia. No one feature is pathognomonic for CS, so diagnosis is often delayed.[13] Sustained hypercortisolism also leads to disorders commonly found in primary care clinics such as hypertension, depression, diabetes, osteoporosis, dyslipidemia, and oligomenorrhea.[12]

Evaluation and diagnosis. There is no single preferred diagnostic test for CS but a careful history should exclude exogenous glucocorticoid intake. Initial screening tests include the late night salivary cortisol test, 24 hour urinary free cortisol test, and dexamethasone suppression test.[14] Interpretation of the test results and further evaluation is best done in consultation with an endocrinologist. When initial screening tests are abnormal, a CRH and desmopressin stimulation tests should be performed with an increase in both plasma ACTH and cortisol on the stimulation tests being indicative of CD.

Once biochemical evidence of CS is found on initial screening tests and stimulation testing, early morning ACTH levels should be measured. Normal to high levels of ACTH suggest CD and warrant a pituitary MRI as the next step.[14] Low ACTH levels suggest an adrenal cause of CS. The presence of an adenoma on MRI helps to establish the diagnosis of CD. Many of the pituitary adenomas are small, and up to 50% may not be seen on MRI. If no tumor is visualized on MRI, further testing with inferior petrosal sinus sampling may be pursued to confirm CD.[14]

Management. Transsphenoidal sinus surgery is the first-line treatment of CD when a pituitary adenoma is found. Rapid reduction of ACTH secretion after surgery leads to CAI in all patients, which requires glucocorticoid replacement going forward. Adenoma recurrence is possible, so lifelong monitoring is indicated.[12]

If an adenoma is not present, surgery is not feasible, or a patient fails to remit after surgery, then radiation or medical therapy can be utilized. Medical therapies such as osilodrostat, metyrapone, and ketoconazole block steroidogenesis in the adrenal gland. These therapies rapidly normalize serum cortisol levels. Pasireotide and cabergoline function to block ACTH centrally and shrink pituitary adenomas but are less effective at normalizing cortisol levels.[14]

Antidiuretic Hormone

ADH is formed in the hypothalamus and stored and released from the posterior pituitary. The main function of ADH is maintenance of plasma tonicity and osmoregulation through alteration of water balance.[15] However, a severe reduction in blood volume shifts the function of ADH primarily to volume regulation, even at the expense of plasma osmolality or tonicity.

Antidiuretic hormone excess: syndrome of inappropriate antidiuretic hormone release

ADH secretion results in concentrated urine and a reduced urine volume. Syndrome of inappropriate antidiuretic hormone release (SIADH) is a condition defined by the unsuppressed release of ADH or its continued action on vasopressin receptors.[15] In most patients with SIADH, ingestion of water does not adequately suppress ADH, and the urine remains concentrated. This leads to water retention, which increases total body water expanding the extracellular fluid volume, which triggers urinary sodium excretion, causing a hypo-osmolar hyponatremia.

Causes. There are multiple causes of SIADH including those related to the CNS, infectious, respiratory, mental health, and medications. In this article, we will only focus on the CNS-related causes of SIADH.

Symptoms. Clinical manifestations of SIADH are typically due to cerebral edema and include fatigue, weakness, nausea, cognitive impairment, headache, gait disturbances and falls, lethargy, seizure, coma, respiratory arrest, and death.[16] Unlike other causes of hyponatremia, SIADH typically does not have peripheral edema, ascites, or orthostasis.

Evaluation/diagnosis. SIADH is difficult to diagnose and can only be made after excluding other causes of hyponatremia including hypothyroidism, renal disease, and adrenal insufficiency. There is no single best test to confirm the diagnosis and is best made with specialty consultation.[16] Assessment of urine osmolality and urine sodium concentration and intravascular volume level is helpful in diagnosing SIADH. The diagnosis of SIADH is suggested by a low plasma osmolality with a high urine osmolality in the setting of hyponatremia. A spot urine sodium greater than 20 mEq/L and low plasma uric acid with a high fractional uric acid excretion are also suggestive of the diagnosis.[16] Brain imaging, particularly when CNS signs or symptoms are present, can be useful to identify specific CNS causes for SIADH.

Treatment. The goal of treatment is slow correction of sodium levels and treatment of any identified underlying etiology. The choice of treatment depends upon the severity of symptoms at presentation and specialty consultation should be utilized in all but very mild hyponatremia.[15] The hallmark of treating SIADH hyponatremia is fluid restriction, although hypertonic saline can be cautiously used in emergent cases of severe hyponatremia. Oral sodium chloride tablets and furosemide can also be used to increase sodium levels and reduce free water.[16] Vasopressin receptor antagonists such as conivaptan (IV) or tolvaptan (oral) are approved for use only in severe persistent SIADH.[16] Other therapies, like lithium or demeclocycline, may also be effective in treating SIADH but are typically only used when other therapies fail.[15,16]

Complications. Severe or acute hyponatremia can cause cerebral edema, and correcting hyponatremia too quickly can lead to osmotic CNS demyelination, a rare but severe neurologic condition, which can result in parkinsonism, quadriparesis, and death.[16]

Antidiuretic hormone deficiency: diabetes insipidus
Background. DI is a rare condition of inadequate production or insensitivity to ADH, which is released in response to changes in plasma osmolality or blood pressure to maintain normal fluid balance via reabsorption of free water at the kidney.[17] Loss of ADH action at the kidney leads to uncontrolled diuresis. Central diabetes insipidus (CDI) includes conditions that affect the release of ADH in the brain whereas nephrogenic diabetes insipidus (NDI) includes conditions that affect the action of ADH on the kidney.[18]

Clinical manifestations. Polyuria, nocturia, and polydipsia are the primary features of DI. Additional symptoms include fatigue, dehydration, and lethargy.[18] Children may exhibit constipation, vomiting, or failure to thrive in addition to the symptoms mentioned earlier. In those with large pituitary tumors triggering DI, headache or visual field defects may arise.[18]

Workup. Initial testing includes confirming polyuria with a 24 hour urine collection. Urine test results should be low for both urine specific gravity and urine osmolality with DI. Elevated plasma osmolality (>300 mOsm/kg) and hypernatremia (Na >145 meq/L) also suggests DI.[19] Performing a water deprivation test while monitoring urine studies has been the standard diagnostic test for DI. The persistence of hypotonic urine in the presence of water deprivation indicates DI.[19] The administration of desmopressin, a synthetic analog of ADH, at the end of the water deprivation test helps to differentiate between CDI and NDI. An increase in urine osmolality upon desmopressin administration (>50%) is consistent with CDI, while an increase of less than 9% is consistent with NDI.

A copeptin level is another diagnostic tool to differentiate between central or nephrogenic causes of DI.[20] Copeptin is contained within the ADH precursor molecule, is easier to measure than ADH, and correlates with levels of ADH. In CDI plasma levels of copeptin are low—even after the presence of stimulation by 3% hypertonic saline. Once the diagnosis of CDI is made, an MRI should be obtained to evaluate for the underlying etiology.[19]

Management. CDI is treated with hydration and desmopressin.[20]

Growth Hormone

GH is a hormone produced by the anterior pituitary gland. GH is responsible for growth regulation during childhood and has metabolic functions and operates as an acute phase stress reactant.[21]

Growth hormone deficiency

Growth hormone deficiency (GHD) is a rare and treatable condition that causes short height in children and metabolic issues in adults. GHD can result from a genetic mutation or damage to the anterior pituitary gland. GHD can be categorized as neonatal, childhood, and adult.

Pediatric growth hormone deficiency: overview. GHD in newborns is a rare disease with a genetic component, but it is also associated with breech presentation and perinatal asphyxia.[22,23] Neonatal GHD can present with isolated GH deficiency but more frequently presents with multiple pituitary hormone deficiencies.[22]

Newborns with GHD present with normal birth length and do not have growth failure until 6 to 12 months of age when the growth velocity deviates from the growth curve.[24] Other common clinical signs include micropenis, hypoglycemia, hypotonia, midline abnormalities, prolonged jaundice, seizure, and global developmental delay.[24,25] Causes of acquired childhood GHD include pituitary tumors, cranial irradiation, and head trauma. Those with GHD typically also display delayed bone age and increased weight-to-height ratios.

Pediatric growth hormone deficiency: evaluation and diagnosis. The diagnosis of GHD in neonates and children is based on clinical findings in combination with laboratory and imaging studies.[24] A random serum GH value of 5 or less to 7 μg/L in the first week of life in combination with a deficiency of other pituitary hormones, hypoglycemia, and/or pituitary radiological abnormalities is sufficient to diagnose GHD in neonates.[24]

In older children, however, GH secretion is highly variable due to pulsatile secretion. Insulin-like growth factor (IGF), insulin-like growth factor binding protein-3 (IGFBP-3) levels, GH stimulation tests, and assessment of bone age are the preferred assessment tests.[23,26,27] If IGF and IGFBP-3 are in the normal range, GHD is extremely unlikely, and no further evaluation is typically required.[23,26,27] Low insulin-like growth factor-1 (IGF-1) and IGFBP-3 with delayed bone age increase the likelihood of GHD, but the diagnosis should typically be confirmed with provocative (stimulation) tests. Commonly used stimulation tests include the glucagon stimulation test, arginine stimulation test, and clonidine stimulation test.[26,28] After the diagnosis of GHD is made, an MRI should be obtained to evaluate for tumors and other structural causes of GHD.[26]

Pediatric growth hormone deficiency: treatment. When diagnosis is confirmed, GH treatment should be initiated. Early replacement therapy leads to more positive outcomes including reduced hypoglycemia, growth recovery, and neurodevelopmental improvements.[24] A multidisciplinary team, including pediatricians, pediatric endocrinologists, geneticists, radiologists, ophthalmologists, and neurologists, should be utilized.

Adult growth hormone deficiency. In adults, GHD is associated with increased visceral adiposity, decreased lean body mass, bone mineral density and exercise capacity, dyslipidemia, insulin resistance, and increased cardiometabolic and fracture risk.[29]

Adult growth hormone deficiency: diagnosis. To avoid overdiagnosis of GHD, it is critical to evaluate only patients at risk for pituitary dysfunction, including those who have had pituitary surgery/mass, radiation therapy, traumatic brain injury, subarachnoid hemorrhage, or childhood onset GHD.[29]

Evaluation for adult growth hormone deficiency. Adults with multiple ($\geq$3) pituitary hormone deficiencies, risk factors for hypopituitarism, and low serum IGF levels are highly likely to have GHD.[29,30] However, the insulin tolerance test (ITT) remains the gold standard test to establish the diagnosis of adult GHD using a peak GH cutoff point of 5 μg/L, but it is laborious and the insulin tolerance test may cause severe hypoglycemia. For adults suspected to have GHD in which the ITT is contraindicated or infeasible, the diagnosis of GH deficiency requires other stimulation tests such as the glucagon-stimulation test and macimorelin test.[29,30]

Adult growth hormone deficiency: treatment. Treatment of adult GH deficiency is done with recombinant human growth hormone (rhGH). GH treatment side effects are related mainly to fluid retention effects and generally respond to dose reductions or cessation of therapy.[30] Treatment with rhGH can also increase blood sugar, complicating underlying diabetes. Treatment with rhGH is contraindicated in patients with most active malignancies and severe diabetic retinopathy.[30]

Growth hormone excess: acromegaly. Acromegaly is a rare chronic disease caused by excessive secretion of GH in adults and typically presents in middle age.[31,32] The most common cause (95% of cases) of acromegaly is a somatotroph adenoma **(Table 1)** of the anterior pituitary.[32] Only about 5% of cases of GH excess occur in children and that condition is called gigantism, as the GH stimulates rapid linear growth. In contrast, adults with acromegaly do not become taller.[32]

Symptoms of acromegaly. The onset and progression of acromegaly symptoms is usually slow, and the average interval from the onset of symptoms until diagnosis is greater than 10 years.[32,33] The typical clinical features in acromegaly include coarsening of facial features, enlarged jaw (macrognathia), enlarged frontal bones and brow protrusion, furrowing of front head, enlargement of the nose and the ears, increased interdental spacing, and thickening of the lips, skin wrinkles, and nasolabial folds.[32] Virtually all patients with acromegaly also have skin thickening and excessive growth of hands and feet due to soft tissue swelling.[32] Soft tissue enlargement in

Table 1
Classification of hormone-secreting pituitary adenomas[6,49,57]

Cell Type	Hormone Secreted	Clinical Syndrome(s)
Corticotroph	ACTH	Cushing's disease
Gonadotroph	LH, FSH	No specific syndrome
Somatotroph	GH	Gigantism, acromegaly
Lactotroph	Prolactin	Hyperprolactinemia
Thyrotroph	TSH	Central hyperthyroidism

acromegaly can cause macroglossia, a deepening of the voice, and obstructive sleep apnea. Unlike other pituitary tumors, tumors associated with acromegaly tend to be large in most patients with 75% of patients having macroadenomas (>10 mm) at diagnosis.[33] Thus, common acromegaly symptoms include headache or visual changes from the tumor mass, as well as those related to GH oversecretion.[33]

Acromegaly also has rheumatologic, cardiovascular, respiratory, neoplastic, neurologic, and metabolic manifestations that negatively impact its prognosis and patient's quality of life. Metabolic consequences of uncontrolled acromegaly include an increased risk of diabetes and impaired glucose tolerance.[32] Some patients have hypertriglyceridemia or hypercalciuria. Most with acromegaly will also have some degree of hypopituitarism as a result of the tumor or ablative therapy.[33,34] Fatigue and weakness can be prominent symptoms. Female individuals with acromegaly can have menstrual dysfunction, galactorrhea, hot flashes, and vaginal atrophy.[32] Male individuals commonly have prostatic enlargement and also commonly present with symptoms of erectile dysfunction, low libido, decreased facial hair growth, and a decrease in testicular volume.[35]

Visceral organs including the thyroid, heart, liver, lungs, prostate, and kidneys enlarge in acromegaly. Cardiovascular abnormalities include hypertension, left ventricular hypertrophy, cardiomyopathy, and heart failure.[34] Increased risk of cancer and colon polyps also occurs in patients diagnosed with acromegaly.[34] Mortality is increased 2 to 3 fold due to cardiovascular, respiratory, and neoplastic disease, although mortality risk acromegaly appears to be reduced by therapy and may be eliminated by cure.[36]

Evaluation and diagnosis. Due to high variability, GH levels are not recommended to diagnose acromegaly.[37,38] The best initial test for the diagnosis is measurement of serum IGF-1.[37,38] A normal serum IGF-1 concentration is strong evidence that the patient does not have acromegaly.[37] A significantly elevated serum IGF-1 concentration in a patient with a typical clinical manifestations of acromegaly is highly suggestive for the diagnosis of acromegaly.[37] However, for cases that are not clear or when IGF-1 levels are equivocal, the diagnosis of acromegaly can be confirmed by an inadequate suppression of serum GH after a glucose load.[38]

For individuals with atypical manifestations of acromegaly, it is still recommended to consider obtaining IGF-1 levels in patients with several of the following conditions: sleep apnea, uncontrolled diabetes, debilitating arthritis, hyperhidrosis, carpal tunnel syndrome, colon polyps, and cardiac failure with hypertension.[38] Following biochemical diagnosis of acromegaly, brain imaging with an MRI should be obtained and formal visual field testing is recommended.[38]

Treatment. Transsphenoidal pituitary surgery is the first-line therapy for patients with acromegaly.[31] The outcome of surgery is very good for microadenomas but up to half of the macroadenomas are not cured surgically and may require postoperative medical therapies.[31,34] Medical therapies include somatostatin receptor ligands, cabergoline, and pegvisomant. Patients with severe sleep apnea or high-output heart failure may also be candidates for preoperative medical therapy to reduce the surgical risk. Also, primary medical therapy has a role for patients without mass effect on the optic chiasm who are unlikely to be cured by surgery. Radiation therapy is usually reserved as a third-line option.[31] Early treatment of acromegaly may improve or resolve diabetes, soft tissue changes, sleep apnea, cardiovascular disease, and neuromuscular disease.[33] Patients should be screened regularly for colon neoplasia (*due to increased colon cancer risk*), even after appropriate acromegaly treatment.[33]

Thyroid-Stimulating Hormone: Pituitary Thyroid Disorders

When evaluating a possible thyroid disorder, it is critical to distinguish primary hyperthyroidism/hypothyroidism due to abnormal functioning of the thyroid gland from central hyperthyroidism/hypothyroidism caused by dysfunction of the pituitary–hypothalamic axis. The pituitary helps control and regulate thyroid function by producing and releasing TSH. Pituitary TSH production is regulated in part by thyrotropin-releasing hormone (TRH), which is secreted from the paraventricular nucleus in the hypothalamus.[39] TRH is transported to the anterior pituitary gland where it regulates the synthesis and release of TSH.[39] TSH then stimulates the synthesis and production of thyroxine (T4) and, to a lesser degree, triiodothyronine (T3) in the thyroid gland.

The diagnosis of central thyroid disorders is based upon clinical manifestations and thyroid function tests. Central hypothyroidism is characterized by a low T4 level and low or normal (noncompensating) TSH level. Central hyperthyroidism is characterized by an elevated T4 and nonsupressed or elevated TSH levels. Pituitary dysfunction is the most common cause of central hyperthyroidism and hyperthyroidism.

Central hyperthyroidism

Central hyperthyroidism is a rare condition in which thyrotoxicosis results from primary overproduction of TSH by the pituitary gland with subsequent thyroid enlargement and hyperfunction. Central hyperthyroidism will have elevated circulating levels of free T4 and T3, and a nonsuppressed serum TSH.[40] Primary hyperthyroidism can be distinguished from central hyperthyroidism because it will have undetectable or very low TSH values with elevated levels of T4 and T3.[40]

The 2 causes of central hyperthyroidism are TSH-producing pituitary tumors (TSHomas) and the syndrome of pituitary resistance to thyroid hormone (PRTH).[40] Both conditions are characterized by clinical thyrotoxicosis, diffuse goiters. In PRTH, the pituitary gland is resistant to the feedback inhibitory effects of circulating thyroid hormones on TSH, while peripheral tissues respond normally, causing patients to experience the toxic peripheral effects of thyroid hormone excess.[40] TSHomas and PRTH can usually be differentiated from one another by measuring the serum alpha-subunit and the TSH response to intravenous TRH or exogenous thyroid hormone. Pituitary imaging studies are also helpful in differentiating the 2 conditions as PRTH is not related to a pituitary tumor and TSHomas are related to a pituitary tumor.[40]

Clinical manifestation: hyperthyroidism. Hyperthyroid symptoms are similar for both primary and central hyperthyroidism and can range from nonsymptomatic, particularly in older patients, to anxiety, emotional lability, cardiac arrhythmias, palpitations, weakness, tremor, myopathy, heat intolerance, increased perspiration, loose stools, menstrual disorders, and unexplained weight loss.[41]

Central hyperthyroidism: evaluation and diagnosis. Initial evaluation of possible central hyperthyroidism should always include at least a TSH and free T4. Other thyroid tests such as T3, free T3, and reverse T3 may also be useful. An elevated T4 and non-supressed or elevated TSH levels are consistent with central hyperthyroidism and necessitate imaging with a brain MRI (preferred) or computed tomographic scan to assess the hypothalamic-pituitary region.

Central hyperthyroidism: treatment. Ideally, initial treatment of central hyperthyroidism should be done in consultation with an endocrinologist. A beta-blocker is typically utilized as soon as the diagnosis is made, to treat adrenergic symptoms. The ideal treatment related to the pituitary gland depends on the etiology. TSHomas (pituitary adenomas) are best treated by transphenoidal surgical removal, and radiotherapy is indicated for inoperable or incompletely resected tumors.[40] Octreotide can be helpful for the medical management of surgical treatment failures for TSHomas and to preoperatively reduce tumor size.[40] PRTH is ideally treated by chronically suppressing TSH secretion with medications including D-thyroxine, triiadothyroacetic acid (TRIAC), octreotide, or bromocriptine.[40] If such therapy is not feasible or ineffective, treatment option includes thyroid ablation with radioiodine or surgery.[40]

Central hypothyroidism

Central hypothyroidism refers to thyroid hormone deficiency due to a disorder of the pituitary, hypothalamus, or hypothalamic–pituitary portal circulation. The most common cause of central hypothyroidism is a pituitary mass.[39,42] Other causes of central hypothyroidism include pituitary or hypothalamic dysfunction due to head trauma, Sheehan syndrome, surgery, radiotherapy, genetic, and infiltrative disease. In patients with hypothyroidism due to pituitary tumors, there may be a deficiency or excess of other pituitary hormones.[43]

Central hypothyroidism: clinical manifestations. The clinical manifestations of central hypothyroidism are similar to those of primary hypothyroidism and common symptoms include fatigue, cold intolerance, weight gain, depressed mood, cognitive changes, cardiac disorders, change in voice, dry skin, constipation, abdominal discomfort, neurosensory changes, edema, myalgias, and life threatening complications such as myxedema.[40] Myxedema is the result of long-standing untreated severe hypothyroidism, and symptoms include altered mental status, hypothermia, lethargy, bradycardia, multisystem organ failure, coma, and even death.[40]

Central hypothyroidism: evaluation and diagnosis. Biochemically, central hypothyroidism is defined by low or low-to-normal TSH concentrations and a low concentration of thyroxine (T4).[40] Initial evaluation for central thyroid disease hypothyroidism in patients is therefore performed by measuring TSH and total or free T4.[44]

It is important to review the prescription and over-the-counter medications the patient is taking as several drugs such as heparin and biotin are known to affect the thyroid testing.[42] Biochemical assessment of the other pituitary hormones should also be performed. Pituitary imaging (MRI preferred) and an ACTH stimulation test to rule out adrenal insufficiency is recommended for all patients with central hypothyroidism.

Central hypothyroidism: treatment. Initial treatment of central hypothyroidism should be done in consultation with an endocrinologist. In rare cases, the central hypothyroidism is transient and resolves without treatment. The main treatment of central hypothyroidism is synthetic levothyroxine.[42–44] Before treating central hypothyroidism with levothyroxine, a thorough evaluation for adrenal insufficiency should also be performed with an ACTH stimulation test. Administration of levothyroxine for central hypothyroidism in patients with unsuspected and/or untreated secondary adrenal insufficiency can precipitate an acute adrenal crisis.[43] Levothyroxine dosing is weight based, and the free T4 is titrated to high normal as serum TSH cannot be used to monitor therapy in those with central hypothyroidism.

Prolactin

Prolactin is involved in breast tissue development and the most common clinical situation for patients with hypoprolactinemia is poor postpartum lactation.[45] Low prolactin levels in this situation should increase the suspicion for Sheehan syndrome and further evaluation for this condition should be performed (see "Sheehan Syndrome" section). Although the evidence is low, use of galactogogues to increase breast milk production may be helpful for lactation insufficiency.[46]

Hyperprolactinemia

Hyperprolactinemia is one of the most common problems in clinical endocrinology and is the most common endocrine disorder of the hypothalamic–pituitary axis.[47,48] Hypogonadism and galactorrhea are well-recognized manifestations of hyperprolactinemia, but it may also have impacts on bone health, metabolism, and the immune system.[48]

Causes of hyperprolactinemia. Physiologic causes of hyperprolactinemia can occur as a part of normal human physiology from pregnancy, breastfeeding, and stress. Other causes of hyperprolactinemia include non-prolactin secreting pituitary disorders, hypothyroidism, chest wall injuries, chronic kidney disease, and medications (*most commonly antipsychotics*).[48]

Prolactinomas are the most common pituitary tumors comprising 40% to 57% of all pituitary adenomas and are the most likely cause of chronic hyperprolactinemia once pregnancy, primary hypothyroidism, and drugs that elevate serum prolactin levels have been excluded.[47,49]

Clinical presentation. There are only a few clinical manifestations of hyperprolactinemia. Women can present with infertility, hypogonadism, galactorrhea, menstrual changes (oligomenorrhea or amenorrhea), osteopenia or osteoporosis, and mass effects of the tumor.[47,50] Male individuals can present with decreased libido, infertility, hypogonadism, gynecomastia, or, rarely, galactorrhea.[49] Postmenopausal women with hyperprolactinemia are asymptomatic unless they have mass effects from the prolactinoma.

Evaluation. Endocrine Society guidelines recommend evaluating for hyperprolactinemia with a single measurement of serum prolactin.[51] Patients with elevated prolactin levels should be referred to endocrinology and evaluated for other causes of hyperprolactinemia such as pregnancy, hypothyroidism, and medications.[51] If no etiology is identified, brain imaging with an MRI should be obtained.[47,51]

Treatment. Following diagnostic evaluation, the next step is to determine whether a patient with hyperprolactinemia has an indication for therapy, such as a macroprolactinoma (tumor >1 cm), hypogonadism, infertility, significant galactorrhea, acne, hirsutism, or headache.[52] Small nonfunctioning adenomas and prolactinomas in asymptomatic patients do not require immediate intervention and can be observed.[52]

The treatment of choice for nearly all patients with hyperprolactinemic disorders is dopamine agonist therapy.[47,52] Dopamine agonists (bromocriptine, pergolide, and cabergoline) are extremely effective in lowering serum prolactin, restoring gonadal function, decreasing tumor size, and improving visual fields.[52] The main limitation to dopamine agonist therapy is side effects that include nausea and dizziness.[52] Cabergoline is the preferred dopamine agonist agent as it appears to be more effective in normalizing prolactin and restoring menses than bromocriptine with better tolerability.[47,52] However, bromocriptine, remains the treatment of choice in hyperprolactinemic women wishing to conceive, due to the paucity of safety data in pregnancy.[47,52] The goals of treatment are to normalize prolactin levels, restore gonadal function, and reduce the effects of chronic hyperprolactinemia.[47]

Follicle-Stimulating Hormone/Luteinizing Hormone: Pituitary Dysfunction

Introduction
LH and FSH are gonadotropins secreted by the anterior pituitary that help regulate gonadal synthesis of various reproductive and sex defining hormones.[53,54] Sexual differentiation, puberty, fertility, and adult sex steroid synthesis depend on this axis being intact.[53,54]

Clinical symptoms
Although gonadotrophic adenomas (see **Table 1**) that secrete LH and FSH rarely produce enough hormone to cause symptoms, patients may present with ovarian hyperstimulation or precocious puberty.[55,56]

Diagnosis/evaluation
If concerned for functional gonadotroph, in addition to FSH and LH levels, is recommended to check a serum alpha subunit level whose present suggests a pituitary origin.[49] Brain imaging should be obtained to evaluate patients with suspected pituitary-related LH/FSH dysfunction.

Treatment
As with all pituitary adenomas, treatment goals include decreasing tumor size to improve mass effect and correcting any hormone imbalances, both of excess and deficiency.[49] Hormonal treatment is not usually necessary for gonadotrophic tumors, but endocrinology should be consulted if hormone levels are significantly abnormal.

CLINICS CARE POINTS

- Suspect Sheehan Syndrome in any postpartum patient with signs of shock.
- Hyperkalemia is a feature of primary adrenal insufficiency, not central adrenal insufficiency.
- No one clinical feature is pathognomonic for Cushing Disease.
- The persistence of hypotonic urine in the presence of water deprivation indicates diabetes insipidus.
- To avoid overdiagnosis of adult growth hormone deficiency, it is important to only evaluate patients with risk factors including prior pitutiary surgery, radiation, subarachnoid hemorrhage, or tramatic brain injury.
- An elevated T4 level paired with non-suppressed TSH is consistent with central hyperthyroidism.

DISCLOSURE

The authors have nothing to disclose.

REFERENCES

1. Karaca Z, Laway BA, Dokmetas HS, et al. Sheehan syndrome. Nat Rev Dis Prim 2016;2:16092.

2. Drummond J.B., Ribeiro-Oliveira A. Jr., Soares B.S., Non-functioning pituitary adenomas. In: Feingold K.R., Anawalt B., Blackman M.R., et al, editors. Endotext internet. South Dartmouth, MA: MDText.com, Inc. 2022. 12-13. Available at: https://www.ncbi.nlm.nih.gov/books/NBK534880/.

3. Kanekar S, Bennett S. Imaging of neurologic conditions in pregnant patients. Radiographics 2016;36(7):2102–22.

4. Matsuzaki S, Endo M, Ueda Y, et al. A case of acute Sheehan's syndrome and literature review: a rare but life-threatening complication of postpartum hemorrhage. BMC Pregnancy Childbirth 2017;17(1):188.

5. Auer MK, Stieg MR, Crispin A, et al. Primary empty sella syndrome and the prevalence of hormonal dysregulation. Dtsch Arztebl Int 2018;115(7):99–105.

6. Melmed S, editor. The pituitary. 4th edition. London: Elsevier; 2017.

7. Houngbadji MSTS, Niang B, Boiro D, et al. Syndrome de résistance à l'Adrénocorticotrophine Hormone (ACTH): à propos d'un cas [Adrenocorticotropic hormone (ACTH) insensitivity syndrome: about a case]. Pan Afr Med J 2018;30:244.

8. Patti G, Guzzeti C, Di Iorgi N, et al. Central adrenal insufficiency in children and adolescents. Best Pract Res Clin Endocrinol Metabol 2018;32(4):425–44.

9. Bitencourt MR, Batista RL, Biscotto I, et al. Central adrenal insufficiency: who, when, and how? From the evidence to the controversies - an exploratory review. Arch Endocrinol Metab 2022;66(4):541–50.

10. Al-Aridi R, Abdelmannan D, Arafah BM. Biochemical diagnosis of adrenal insufficiency: the added value of dehydroepiandrosterone sulfate measurements. Endocr Pract 2011;17(2):261–70.

11. Dineen R, Thompson CJ, Sherlock M. Adrenal crisis: prevention and management in adult patients. Ther Adv Endocrinol Metab 2019;10. 2042018819848218.

12. Reincke M, Fleseriu M. Cushing syndrome: a review. JAMA 2023;330(2):170–81.

13. Sharma ST, Nieman LK, Feelders RA. Cushing's syndrome: epidemiology and developments in disease management. Clin Epidemiol 2015;7:281–93.

14. Fleseriu M, Ieseriu M, Auchus R, et al. Consensus on diagnosis and management of Cushing's disease: a guideline update. Lancet Diabetes Endocrinol 2021; 9(12):847–75.

15. Yasir M, Mechanic OJ. Syndrome of inappropriate antidiuretic hormone secretion. In: StatPearls [internet]. Treasure Island (FL): StatPearls Publishing; 2023. Available at: https://www.ncbi.nlm.ni.h.gov/books/NBK507777/.

16. Adrogué HJ, Tucker BM, Madias NE. Diagnosis and management of hyponatremia: a review. JAMA 2022;328(3):280–91.

17. Park EJ, Kwon TH. A minireview on vasopressin-regulated aquaporin-2 in kidney collecting duct cells. Electrolyte Blood Press 2015;13(1):1–6.

18. Hui C, Khan M, Khan Suheb MZ, et al. Diabetes insipidus. In: StatPearls [Internet]. Treasure Island (FL): StatPearls Publishing; 2023.

19. Christ-Crain M, Gaisl O. Diabetes insipidus. Presse Med 2021;50(4):104093.

20. Refardt J, Winzeler B, Christ-Crain M. Copeptin and its role in the diagnosis of diabetes insipidus and the syndrome of inappropriate antidiuresis. Clin Endocrinol (Oxf) 2019;91(1):22–32.

21. Vanderkuur JA, Butch ER, Waters SB, et al. Signaling molecules involved in coupling growth hormone receptor to mitogen-activated protein kinase activation. Endocrinology 1997;138(10):4301–7.

22. Binder G, Weber K, Rieflin N, et al. Diagnosis of severe growth hormone deficiency in the newborn. Clin Endocrinol 2020;93:305–11.

23. Hage C, Gan HW, Ibba A, et al. Advances in differential diagnosis and management of growth hormone deficiency in children. Nat Rev Endocrinol 2021;17(10): 608–24.

24. Stagi S, Tufano M, Chiti N, et al. M. Management of Neonatal Isolated and Combined Growth Hormone Deficiency: Current Status. Int J Mol Sci 2023;24(12): 10114.

25. Xatzipsalti M, Voutetakis A, Stamoyannou L, et al. Congenital hypopituitarism: various genes, various phenotypes. Horm Metab Res 2019;51:81–90.

26. Growth Hormone Research Society. Consensus guidelines for the diagnosis and treatment of growth hormone (GH) deficiency in childhood and adolescence: summary statement of the GH Research Society. GH Research Society. J Clin Endocrinol Metab 2000;85(11):3990–3.

27. Bancos I, Algeciras-Schimnich A, Grebe SK, et al. Evaluation of variables influencing the measurement of insulin-like growth factor-1. Endocr Pract 2014; 20(5):421–6.

28. Yackobovitch-Gavan M, Lazar L, Diamant R, et al. Diagnosis of growth hormone deficiency in children: the efficacy of glucagon versus clonidine stimulation test. Horm Res Paediatr 2020;93(7–8):470–6.

29. Tritos NA, Biller BMK. Current concepts of the diagnosis of adult growth hormone deficiency. Rev Endocr Metab Disord 2021;22(1):109–16.

30. Yuen KCJ, Biller BMK, Radovick S, et al. American association of clinical endocrinologists and american college of endocrinology guidelines for management of growth hormone deficiency in adults and patients transitioning from pediatric to adult care. Endocr Pract 2019;25(11):1191–232.

31. Ershadinia N, Tritos NA. Diagnosis and treatment of acromegaly: an update. Mayo Clin Proc 2022;97(2):333–46.

32. Vilar L, Vilar CF, Lyra R, et al. Acromegaly: clinical features at diagnosis. Pituitary 2017;20(1):22–32.

33. Molitch ME. Clinical manifestations of acromegaly. Endocrinol Metab Clin N Am 1992;21:597.

34. Capatina C, Wass JA. 60 years of neuroendocrinology: acromegaly. J Endocrinol 2015;226(2):T141–60.

35. Salvio G, Martino M, Balercia G, et al. Acromegaly and male sexual health. Rev Endocr Metab Disord 2022;23(3):671–8.

36. Sherlock M, Reulen RC, Alonso AA, et al. ACTH deficiency, higher doses of hydrocortisone replacement, and radiotherapy are independent predictors of mortality in patients with acromegaly. J Clin Endocrinol Metab 2009;94:4216.

37. Akirov A, Masri-Iraqi H, Dotan I, et al. The biochemical diagnosis of acromegaly. J Clin Med 2021;10.

38. Katznelson L, Laws ER, Melmed S, et al. Acromegaly: an endocrine society clinical practice guideline. J Clin Endocrinol Metab 2014;99:3933.

39. Kondo Y, Ozawa A, Kohno D, et al. The hypothalamic paraventricular nucleus is the center of the hypothalamic-pituitary-thyroid axis for regulating thyroid hormone levels. Thyroid 2022;32:105.

40. McDermott MT, Ridgway EC. Central hyperthyroidism. Endocrinol Metab Clin N Am 1998;27(1):187–203.

41. Boelaert K, Torlinska B, Holder RL, et al. Older subjects with hyperthyroidism present with a paucity of symptoms and signs: a large cross-sectional study. J Clin Endocrinol Metab 2010;95(6):2715–26.

42. Chaker L, Bianco AC, Jonklaas J, et al. Hypothyroidism. Lancet 2017;390(10101): 1550–62.

43. Persani L. Clinical review: Central hypothyroidism: pathogenic, diagnostic, and therapeutic challenges. J Clin Endocrinol Metab 2012;97:3068.
44. Persani L, Cangiano B, Bonomi M. The diagnosis and management of central hypothyroidism in 2018. Endocr Connect 2019;8(2):R44–54.
45. Karayazi Atıcı Ö, Govindrajan N, Lopetegui-González I, et al. Prolactin: A hormone with diverse functions from mammary gland development to cancer metastasis. Semin Cell Dev Biol 2021;114:159–70.
46. Foong SC, Tan ML, Foong WC, et al. Oral galactagogues (natural therapies or drugs) for increasing breast milk production in mothers of non-hospitalised term infants. Cochrane Database Syst Rev 2020;5(5):CD011505.
47. Mah PM, Webster J. Hyperprolactinemia: etiology, diagnosis, and management. Semin Reprod Med 2002;20(4):365–74.
48. Samperi I, Lithgow K, Karavitaki N. Hyperprolactinaemia. J Clin Med 2019;8(12):2203.
49. Lake MG, Krook LS, Cruz SV. Pituitary adenomas: an overview. Am Fam Physician 2013;88(5):319–27.
50. Bayrak A, Saadat P, Mor E, et al. Pituitary imaging is indicated for the evaluation of hyperprolactinemia. Fertil Steril 2005;84(1):181–5.
51. Melmed S, Casanueva FF, Hoffman AR, et al. Endocrine society. diagnosis and treatment of hyperprolactinemia: an endocrine society clinical practice guideline. J Clin Endocrinol Metab 2011;96(2):273–88.
52. Biller BM. Hyperprolactinemia. Int J Fertil Women's Med 1999;44(2):74–7. PMID: 10338264.
53. Ojeda SR, Ma YJ. Glial-neuronal interactions in the neuroendocrine control of mammalian puberty: facilitatory effects of gonadal steroids. J Neurobiol 1999;40(4):528–40.
54. Ruwanpura SM, McLachlan RI, Meachem SJ. Hormonal regulation of male germ cell development. J Endocrinol 2010;205(2):117–31.
55. Molitch ME. Nonfunctioning pituitary tumors and pituitary incidentalomas. Endocrinol Metab Clin N Am 2008;37(1):151–xi.
56. Ntali G, Capatina C, Grossman A, et al. Clinical review: functioning gonadotroph adenomas. J Clin Endocrinol Metab 2014;99(12):4423–33.
57. Zargar AH, Laway BA, Masoodi SR, et al. Clinical and endocrine aspects of pituitary tumors. Saudi Med J 2004;25(10):1428–32.

Multiple Endocrine Neoplasia Type 1, Type 2A, and Type 2B

Leslie A. Greenberg, MD, FAAFP

KEYWORDS

- Multiple endocrine neoplasia • MEN 1 • MEN 2A • MEN 2B

KEY POINTS

- Multiple endocrine neoplasia Type 1 causes endocrine tumors affecting parathyroid glands, the gastrointestinal tract, andthe anterior pituitary gland.
- Multiple endocrine neoplasia Type 2A is a genetic syndrome and causes medullary thyroid cancer (MTC) and may also cause pheochromocytomas, primary hyperparathyroidism, cutaneous lichen amyloidosis, and Hirschsprung's disease.
- Multiple endocrine neoplasia Type 2B is a rare genetic mutation that causes MTC and can also cause pheochromocytomas, benign ganglioneuromas of the digestive tract, face, and eyelid and skeletal abnormalities.

INTRODUCTION

Multiple endocrine neoplasia is a group of conditions caused by genetic mutations. The specific gene mutation dictates which disease process occurs (Multiple endocrine neoplasia type 1 [MEN1], Multiple endocrine neoplasia type 2A [MEN2A], or Multiple endocrine neoplasia type 2B [MEN2B]), which endocrine tumors are formed, and even the age tumors are expected. Suspicion of these entities is paramount to assist with information gathering and prognosis. Detailed family history, personal symptom history, examination, laboratory tests, and imaging are crucial to help diagnose the patient and make an appropriate surveillance plan.

MULTIPLE ENDOCRINE NEOPLASIA TYPE I
Introduction

MEN1 is a rare genetic neuroendocrine syndrome where the same individual or related individuals of the same family have endocrine tumors affecting primarily the parathyroid glands, diffuse neuroendocrine tissues of the gastroenteropancreatic tract, and

Department of Family and Community Medicine, University of Nevada Reno School of Medicine, 745 West Moana Lane, Reno, NV 89509, USA
E-mail address: lgreenberg@med.unr.edu

Prim Care Clin Office Pract 51 (2024) 483–494
https://doi.org/10.1016/j.pop.2024.03.006
0095-4543/24/Published by Elsevier Inc.

primarycare.theclinics.com

the anterior pituitary gland. MEN1 is a highly penetrant autosomal dominant trait. Less than 10% of MEN1 cases are considered de novo. More than 1500 different germline and somatic mutations have been reported in the MEN1 gene locus.[1] MEN1 is caused by germline heterozygous loss-of-function mutations in the tumor suppressor gene MEN1, located on chromosome 11 (11q13.1), which encodes the protein menin. Germline MEN1 mutations must coexist with the loss of the unaffected MEN1 allele to cause tumorigenesis.

Clinical Features

No simple definition of MEN1 can encompass all index cases or all families. It affects individuals aged from 5 years to 82 years.[1] MEN1 causes a combination of over 20 different endocrine and nonendocrine tumors. MEN1-related cancers have no effective prevention or cure because the principal cancer host organs (pancreas, duodenum, and lungs) are difficult to screen for early tumors and are not appropriate for ablative or excisional surgery. Thus, even in the presence of a positive genetic test, prophylactic tumor prevention is often not possible.

Parathyroid tumors

The most common feature of MEN1 is primary hyperparathyroidism (PHPT) with hypercalcemia diagnosed in individuals aged between 20 years and 30 years. More than 94% of patients will have clinical or biochemical manifestations of PHPT by the fifth decade of life.[2] Parathyroid tumors are multiglandular and asymmetric.[3] Hyperparathyroidism can present with tiredness, nausea, vomiting, kidney stones, and bone pain. Bone density in women with MEN1 and hyperparathyroidism is often low by age 35.[4]

Neuroendocrine tumors

Duodenopancreatic neuroendocrine tumors (NETs) are present with symptomatic gastrinomas (Zollinger Ellison syndrome) or insulinomas but may also be asymptomatic due to a non-secreting tumor. Hypergastrinemia may cause excessive gastric acid production, peptic ulcers, gastric perforations, and diarrhea. The majority of gastrinomas is in the duodenum and is often multiple and less than 0.5 cm in diameter. MEN 1-related gastrinomas usually have a malignant component and half have metastasized before diagnosis.[5] Gastrinomas represent more than half of all duodenopancreatic NETs in patients with MEN1.[6]

Insulinomas present with Whipple's triad (hypoglycemia symptoms, low blood sugar, and resolution of symptoms when glucose is increased) and may lead to recurrent hypoglycemia attacks, which may induce seizures. Glucagonomas, vasoactive intestinal peptide tumors (VIPomas), and somatostatinomas are rare. VIPomas present with the constellation of watery diarrhea, hypokalemia, and achlorhydria.

Pituitary tumors

Clinical manifestations of pituitary tumors are related to the hormones secreted by the tumor: 60% secrete prolactin, 25% growth hormone, and 5% corticotropin. Enlarging pituitary tumors can compress the optic chiasm and cause visual disturbances and is the most common presenting symptom in a patient with a nonfunctioning adenoma. Diffuse headaches are the second most common neurologic symptom because of sellar expansion. Prolactinoma is the most common pituitary adenoma followed by somatotropinoma. Prolactinomas present with oligomenorrhea, amenorrhea, and galactorrhea in women and sexual dysfunction, impotence, infertility or (rarely) gynecomastia in men. Excess growth hormone presents with acromegaly. Adrenocortical involvement is usually asymptomatic because the tumors are non-functional.

Thymic NETs are often aggressive; malignant tumors that do not secrete hormones and are usually detected in imaging studies. Nonfunctioning tumors cause no clinical symptoms or biochemical changes.[6,7]

Diagnosis

Definitive diagnosis is gene testing. Results reveal a mutation in the MEN1 gene located on chromosome 11 (11q13.1). MEN1 is clinically diagnosed by the presence of tumors in at least 2 of the 3 main MEN 1 affected organs: parathyroids, endocrine pancreas, and anterior pituitary or if an individual has 1 of these tumors and a first-degree relative has MEN 1.

To properly diagnose MEN1, one should obtain family history of endocrinopathies, tumors, and cancers. A history should also include inquiries about diarrhea, steatorrhea, nausea, diabetes, erythematous rash, vomiting, amenorrhea, galactorrhea, sexual dysfunction, impotence, infertility, kidney stones, bone pain, and symptoms of hypoglycemia. Hyperparathyroidism can present with tiredness, nausea, vomiting, kidney stones, and bone pain. Prolactinomas can cause oligomenorrhea, amenorrhea, and galactorrhea. VIPomas present with the constellation of watery diarrhea, hypokalemia, and achlorhydria.[7,8]

A physical examination for non-endocrine features includes lipomas, facial angiofibromas, histiocytofibromas, or collagenomas.

Once MEN1 diagnosis has been made, a multidisciplinary team is needed: endocrinology, gastroenterology, oncology, pathology, radiology, nuclear medicine, genetics, and endocrine tumor surgeon.

Consider MEN1 genetic testing with familial isolated hyperparathyroidism, parathyroid hyperplasia, or adenoma less than 40 years of age, recurrent or multiglandular PHPT at any age, gastrinoma, or multifocal gastroduodenopancreatic neuroendocrine tumor, bronchial or thymic NET, or relative with known MEN1 pathogenic mutation. First-degree relatives should be offered genetic screening for MEN1 germline mutations because there is a 50% risk of passing on the MEN1 gene mutation. If positive, then complete screening for MEN1-associated tumors should be offered.[7,8]

Further Evaluation

If patient has laboratory proven MEN1 gene mutation and is asymptomatic, then:

- Screen for tumors with annual biochemical evaluation- calcium, parathyroid hormone (PTH), prolactin, Insulin-like growth factor-1 (IGF-1), Chromogranin A, fasting glucose, insulin, gastrin, vasointestinal polypeptide (VIP), and pancreatic polypeptide
- Routine imaging of MRI pituitary and abdominal imaging (MRI or computed tomography [CT]) every 1 year to 3 years and thymic and lung CT or MRI every 1 year to 2 years.[6]
- Screening should begin in early childhood and be repeated throughout life.

In laboratory proven MEN1 gene mutation and symptomatic, the authors further divide it by tumor type.

Parathyroid Tumors

To test for hyperparathyroidism obtain laboratories to include serum calcium and PTH. If abnormal add albumin, creatinine, phosphate, 25-OH Vitamin D, and urinary calcium excretion. Imaging includes a neck ultrasound, dual X-ray absorptiometry (DEXA), and renal ultrasound with abnormal laboratories .[4]

Neuroendocrine Tumors

For gastroduodenopancreatic NETs screening laboratories should include gastrin, glucagon, VIP, pancreatic polypeptide, insulin, and chromogranin A. Imaging for all gastroduodenopancreatic NETs should include abdominal CT or MRI or endoscopic ultrasound annually or endoscopy to search for intraluminal gastric NETs every 3 years. Patients with glucagonoma may present with a characteristic rash of necrotizing migratory erythema and new onset diabetes. For these reasons patients obtain glucagon level. For patients with VIPoma, obtain VIP level. For somatostatinoma, serum plasma somatostatin concentration should be obtained. For evaluation of insulinoma, obtain glucose and insulin levels. If patients are symptomatic and there is suspicion for insulinoma, the most reliable test is a supervised 72 hour fast, in which increased plasma insulin concentration is present with hypoglycemia. An elevated circulating C-peptide and proinsulin concentrations help establish the diagnosis.[7]

Pituitary Tumors

Corticotroph adenomas usually cause Cushing's disease and are best diagnosed with an elevated adrenocorticotropic hormone (ACTH) and cortisol level. Prolactinomas are best diagnosed with a prolactin level. For evaluation of a non-functioning and gonadotropin-secreting adenomas obtain prolactin, insulin-like growth factor 1 (IGF1), and other pituitary hormones (leutinising hormone, follicle stimulating hormone, and human chorionic gonadotropin hormone) if there are symptoms orr signs. For somatotropinoma, the single best test for the diagnosis of acromegaly is serum IGF1. For cortisol-secreting tumor obtain late-night salivary cortisol level, an overnight 1 mg dexamethasone test, 24-hour urinary-free cortisol, and ACTH. For thyroid stimulating hormone (TSH)-secreting tumor, obtain TSH and free T4.

Imaging for adrenocortical tumors includes abdominal CT or MRI. For aldosterone-secreting tumor obtain aldosterone to renin ratio. For adrenocortical carcinoma testosterone, DHEA-S and delta 4-androstenedione is obtained.[7]

Treatment

Before making a treatment plan regarding MEN1 tumors, assess if tumors are metastatic.

Parathyroid tumors
Definitive treatment of parathyroid tumors is surgical resection (subtotal or total parathyroidectomy, with or without autotransplantation of parathyroid tissue). Concurrent transcervical thymectomy is suggested at the time of parathyroidectomy surgery to remove a future endocrine tumor source.[6]

Neuroendocrine tumors
Gastrinoma treatment includes proton pump inhibitors with or without histamine H2 receptor antagonist or surgical excision of gastrinomas. Most patients with MEN1 will have multiple small submucosal duodenal gastrinomas making surgical management difficult. Somatostatin analogs prevent severe and life-threatening morbidity in MEN1 by decreasing the oversecretion of enteropancreatic hormones.[8] Early surgical or pharmacologic intervention is warranted. Treatment of symptomatic adrenal hormone-secreting tumors, insulinomas, carcinoids, glucagonomas, and VIPomas is surgical. Post-treatment follow-up imaging for thymic or bronchopulmonary NETs includes a chest CT or MRI.[7]

Pituitary tumors

Prolactinomas are treated medically with dopamine agonists or surgical resection. Somatotrophinomas are medically treated with octreotide or lanreotide or transsphenoidal surgical hypophysectomy. Radiotherapy is reserved for residual unresectable pituitary tumor. For follow-up on pituitary adenomas, obtain an annual plasma prolactin and IGF-1 levels and a pituitary MRI every 3 years.

Complications

The NETs can cause gastric ulcers with perforation and hypoglycemia. PHPT can cause severe bone demineralization, osteoporosis, hypercalcemia, and urolithiasis-related renal complications. Post-surgical complications include pancreatic fistulas, delayed gastric emptying, bile leakage, chyle leakage after Whipple procedure, or resultant hypocalcemia from parathyroidectomy. Metastatic disease is common with innumerable complications. Untreated patients with MEN1 have a decreased life expectancy with a 50% probability of death by the age of 50.[6]

MULTIPLE ENDOCRINE NEOPLASIA TYPE 2

Multiple endocrine neoplasia type 2 (MEN2) is an autosomal dominant genetic syndrome that occurs because of a germline variant in the rearranged during transfection RET proto-oncogene. Hyperactivation of the receptor leads to induction of downstream signals responsible for oncogenesis. It has malignant potential. The prevalence of MEN2A is 13 per million to 24 per million[9] and 1 per million to 2 per million for MEN2B.[10,11] There are nearly 200 known mutations resulting in a gain-of-function that encodes for a constitutively activated transmembrane RET tyrosine kinase receptor.

MEN2 is classified into 3 subtypes: MEN2A (70%–80%), MEN2B (5%), and familial medullary thyroid carcinoma (10%–20%). De novo variants are rare in MEN2A (6%–9%), but common in MEN2B (>90%).[12–14] The genetic mutations causing MEN2 are a relatively new scientific finding: RET proto-oncogene is on chromosome 10 (10q11.12) and contains 21 exons and was discovered as an oncogene in 1985.[15–17]

The cardinal manifestation in MEN2 is MTC, either isolated or associated with other endocrine tumors or typical features. Mortality in MEN2 is directly related to MTC. This receptor activation can cause medullary thyroid carcinoma, pheochromocytoma, primary hyperparathyroidism, cutaneous lichen amyloidosis, and Hirschsprung's disease.[11]

MULTIPLE ENDOCRINE NEOPLASIA TYPE 2A
Introduction

MEN2A is subdivided into 4 phenotypes.

1. Classical MEN2A associated with MTC, pheochromocytoma and PHPT.
2. MEN2A associated with cutaneous lichen amyloidosis.
3. MEN2A associated with Hirschsprung's disease.
4. Familial MTC that only results in MTC.

Classical MEN2A is the most common phenotype. Overall MEN2A is characterized by MTC 100%, 35% primary PHTH, and 50% with pheochromocytomas.[15] Pheochromocytomas are a chromaffin cell tumor that secretes excess catecholamine that can be detected as elevated levels of plasma free metanephrines and normetanephrines. For smaller pheochromocytomas, there is a surgical window of opportunity to perform an endoscopic subtotal or tissue-sparing adrenalectomy, aiming to preserve a minimum of 15% to 30% of adrenal tissue to circumvent steroid dependency and

Addisonian crisis.[18] If primary hyperparathyroidism is present, it is more often associated with a 634-RET mutation and there's multiglandular disease.

MTC develops after C-cell hyperplasia and is usually the first manifestation of the syndrome.[19] MTC is a rare calcitonin-producing tumor arising from the thyroid parafollicular C cells. The surgical window of opportunity to avoid metastatic MTC is open if serum calcitonin levels remain within normal limits. Once MTC metastasizes, it usually spreads to local and regional lymph nodes, and more distantly to lung, liver, and bone. Decreased survival in MTC is correlated with the stage at the time of diagnosis. Current practice is to perform prophylactic thyroidectomy before development of MTC in at-risk patients.[20]

MEN2A with cutaneous lichen amyloidosis presents with amyloid deposits in the upper dermis in the scapular region. MEN2A with Hirschsprung's disease often presents with gastrointestinal symptoms within the first year of life of bilious emesis, abdominal distension, and failure to pass meconium or stool. Familial MTC in which MTC patients have multiple family members with MTC and none have pheochromocytomas or primary hyperparathyroidism.[21]

Clinical Features

Most MEN2A patients are not symptomatic at MTC diagnosis.[11] Excess calcitonin in MTC may cause diarrhea and flushing. If posterior thyroid tumors are present, hoarseness, dysphagia, or respiratory distress may be a presenting symptom.

Pheochromocytoma is prevalent in 17% to 42% of MEN2A cases and can be the first manifestation, but in most cases the diagnosis of pheochromocytoma is made simultaneously or after MTC. Patients may present with hypertension or hypotension, palpitations, sweating, and headaches because of the adrenergic secretory status of the tumor and hypertensive crisis is rare.[22]

The median age of the cutaneous manifestation in cutaneous lichen amyloidosis is 13 year old.[21] Consider MEN2A in pediatric patients aged less than 1 year with Hirschsprung's, either short or long-segment disease.

Evaluation

Obtain family history of MTC, PHPT, or pheochromocytoma. Inquire about hoarseness, dysphagia, respiratory distress, hypertension, hypotension, palpitations, sweating, headaches, itchy scaly rash on the upper back, diarrhea, or flushing.

Physical examination of neck is done to assess for thyroid mass or lymphadenopathy. Cutaneous lichen amyloidosis may present as an itchy scaly rash on the upper back that improves with sun exposure and worsens during stress.[22]

In terms of laboratory analysis, a DNA analysis for RET germline mutation, calcitonin, CEA, PTH, calcium, and neck ultrasound should be obtained.

RET mutational gene analysis starting with codons 10 and 11 should be performed on index case in presence of MTC or pheochromocytoma or in an asymptomatic first-degree relative of a known MEN2A mutation carrier.[23] Ninety eight percent of MEN2A patients have a RET mutation in either exons 10 or 11 with the most frequent mutation involving exon 11 codon 634.[15]

If suspicious for pheochromocytoma, if the RET genetic test returns positive, further surveillance laboratories are indicated. These surveillance laboratories include catecholamines and a plasma or urine metanephrines and normetanephrines. Catecholamines are not a reliable marker because the inconsistent rate of secretion. A 4-time increase of catecholamine plasma concentration is rarely seen in a patient without pheochromocytomas. If there's inconclusive biochemistry, a clonidine suppression test is done.[24]

To decrease factitious results, obtain calcitonin during fasting, before contrast imaging, and avoid heavy meals or alcohol the night before. Serum calcitonin, the hallmark of MTC, is used for early detection and diagnosis and prognosis after total thyroidectomy (TT). High serum calcitonin (>100 pg/mL) is correlated with MTC presence. Metastasis can be present with calcitonin greater than 20 pg/mL. Carcinoembryonic antigen (CEA) is another serologic marker of MTC and is elevated in more than 50% of patients with MTC. CEA values greater than 100 ng/mL suggest extensive local adenopathy or distant metastases.[25]

Treatment

In all patients with MEN2A, pheochromocytoma must be excluded before any surgical intervention. If a pheochromocytoma exists, preoperative pharmacologic alpha-adrenergic blockade may be needed before surgery. Surgical excision of pheochromocytoma should be performed before thyroidectomy or parathyroidectomy when diagnosis of pheochromocytoma and MTC or hyperparathyroidism is synchronous. TT is the surgery of choice for MTC because the RET mutation often causes multiple tumors. If parathyroid glands are devascularized during TT, parathyroid tissue can be auto transplanted to the non-dominant forearm or in the sternocleidomastoid muscle. Parathyroid glands that have been manipulated may not become functional until 2 months postoperatively, so frequent calcium level monitoring and adequate calcium replacement is essential. Parathyroid gland transplantation to the forearm is also helpful if subsequent hyperparathyroidism occurs in the remaining gland and the gland needs removal. This allows for the excision to be done under local anesthesia without re-entering the neck.[26]

Surveillance

After TT, calcitonin doubling time has important prognostic value and documents metastatic MTC. Genetic and pre-conception counseling is important as an offspring has a 50% chance of inheriting the mutated gene.[23]

Annual surveillance laboratories, starting at the age of 8, are necessary when MEN2A hyperparathyroidism is suspected: calcium, albumin, PTH, phosphate, and urinary calcium. After parathyroidectomy, monitor serum calcium and creatinine annually and bone density by DEXA scan every 18 months to 24 months.[3]

Complications

Long standing hyperparathyroidism can cause bone demineralization with resulting osteoporosis and increased fracture risk. MTC metastatic disease has complications related to future metastectomies or side effects from medications intended to shrink metastatic lesions called multikinase and selective RET kinase inhibitors. These medication side effects are diarrhea (56%), rash (45%), nausea (33%), hypertension (32%), and headaches (26%).[27] Surgical complications from parathyroidectomy or TT include hypocalcemia and injury to the recurrent laryngeal nerve with resulting hoarseness. Complications from bilateral adrenalectomy can cause adrenal insufficiency and difficulty autoregulating corticosteroids.

MULTIPLE ENDOCRINE NEOPLASIA TYPE 2B
Introduction

MEN2B is associated with MTC, pheochromocytomas, ganglioneuromas of the digestive tract, face, and eyelid and skeletal abnormalities. MEN2B patients do not have hyperparathyroidism. MEN2B is commonly caused by a RET mutation in codon 918 and 883 in approximately 95% and 5%, respectively. 94% of MEN2B patients are de novo variants.[28] The earlier identification of MEN2B is helpful so that early TT is performed, and metastatic disease is avoided. Early clinical recognition of MEN2B is difficult because the rarity of the condition, the rare familial link, and the development of aggressive childhood cancer. The International RET Mutation Consortium correlated the specific mutation with clinical aggressiveness of hereditary MTC and published guidelines for the timing of prophylactic thyroidectomy.[29]

Clinical Features

Clinical features show that 100% have MTC, 50% have pheochromocytomas, and specific body features. To improve prognosis of MEN2B patient it is imperative to be aware of the extra-endocrine signs of this rare syndrome. The extra-endocrine features that increase suspicion of MEN2B are.[13]

1. Multiple ganglioneuromas that appear as small soft sessile painless papules 2 mm to 7 mm yellow to white on the tongue (62%) (**Fig. 1**) and lips (53%).
2. When intestinal autonomic ganglion dysfunction occurs, this can lead to constipation and mega colon.
3. Marfanoid habitus is prevalent with joint laxity (73%), pes cavus (38%), hypotonia (27%), pectus excavatum (26%), and scoliosis (9%).
4. Corneal nerve hypertrophy (45%), tearless crying (40%), and neuromas on the eyelid or conjunctiva (19%).

Not all extra-endocrine features are present at birth but become recognizable during the first decade of life. The clinical picture and behavior of MEN2B-related pheochromocytomas is like that of MEN2A-related pheochromocytomas.

Evaluation

Look for the physical examination findings in children. If MEN2B is missed, most die from metastatic MTC before adulthood. Physical examination is done to evaluate

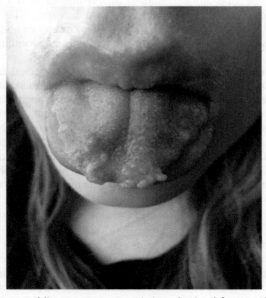

Fig. 1. Benign tongue and lip neuromas. Permission obtained from patient.

for bumps on the eyelids, tongue or lips, marfanoid habitus, long arms, pes cavus, hypotonia, striae, easy bruising, pectus excavatum, and scoliosis. If MTC is present and impinges on other structures, the patient may have neck discomfort, difficulty swallowing or breathing, or hoarse voice. Flushing or diarrhea can also occur because of excess calcitonin secreted by the parafollicular C cells that cause MTC.[13,28,29]

Evaluation should also include laboratory work consisting of germline RET mutation analysis of exons 15 and 16, calcitonin, CEA, calcium, PTH, plasma (or urine) metanephrines, and normetanephrines. To decrease factitious results, draw lab for calcitonin while fasting, before contrast imaging, and avoid heavy meals or alcohol the night before. The CEA is elevated in MTC and is obtained at the same time as calcitonin. Plasma or urine metanephrines and normetanephrines are measured for evaluation of pheochromocytomas. Catecholamines are not a reliable marker because of the inconsistent rate of secretion.[27,28]

Other diagnostics includes a neck ultrasound to evaluate for thyroid lesions and surrounding lymph nodes. If gastrointestinal symptoms are present, rectal biopsy can lead to the diagnosis of intestinal ganglioneuromatosis.[30]

Treatment

TT with central lymph node dissection is the mainstay of treatment timing of TT may be before first birthday in patients with known mutation of 918. Prompt TT is the only cure of MTC and should be performed at an MTC high-volume center as the surgery is delicate and the primary surgery is nearly their only chance for longevity. Postoperatively, the TSH should be within the normal range with routine thyroid replacement. TSH suppression is not needed and no radioactive iodine treatment needed.[28]

Surveillance

For MTC, postoperatively repeat calcitonin after 3 months to allow for "wash out." This value is the calcitonin nadir–the new calcitonin baseline. At 6 months post-operative visit obtain neck ultrasound, calcitonin, and CEA. From this point on there is long-term monitoring with calcitonin, CEA, neck ultrasound, and plasma (or urine) metanephrines and normetanephrines.[13,25,26]

Long-term monitoring for pheochromocytomas is important. In cases of elevated plasma or urine metanephrines and normetanephrines, adrenal MRI or CT is recommended. CT is the preferable imaging as it provides higher resolution and sensitivity for small adrenal tumors. CT has 93% to 100% sensitivity in detecting intraadrenal tumors greater than 0.5 cm. Sensitivity of 90% for localizing extra adrenal pheochromocytomas greater than 1 cm.[31] Patient with pheochromocytomas require alpha blockade with or without beta blockade before and during surgery. Adrenal-sparing removal of the pheochromocytoma is the preferred surgery. Laparoscopic adrenalectomy or retroperitoneoscopic adrenalectomy is now the favored surgical approach. Cancer markers calcitonin and CEA should also be followed.[32]

Genetic and pre-conception counseling is imperative as MEN2B patients are usually diagnosed before reproductive age and there's a 50% risk of passing the same RET gene mutation to their offspring.[23]

Complications

The most common complication of MEN2B is metastatic MTC due to the de novo nature of the condition and delay in TT. MTC metastatic disease has complications related to future metastectomies or side effects from medications intended to shrink metastatic lesions called multikinase and selective RET kinase inhibitors. These medication side effects are diarrhea (56%), rash (45%), nausea (33%), hypertension (32%)

and headaches (26%).[27] Surgical complications from total thyroidectomy include transient hypocalcemia after TT and injury to the recurrent laryngeal nerve with resulting hoarseness. Complications from bilateral adrenalectomy can cause adrenal insufficiency and difficulty in autoregulating corticosteroids.[32]

CLINICS CARE POINTS

- MEN1 can cause 20 different endocrine and nonendocrine tumors.
- MEN1 individuals often have relatives with endocrine tumors.
- MEN1 diagnosis is caused by a mutation on chromosome 11 and involves annual surveillance laboratories and imaging to diagnose tumors.
- MEN2A causes MTC, pheochromocytoma, primary hyperparathyroidism, cutaneous lichen amyloidosis, and Hirschsprung's disease.
- MEN2A often requires surgical excision of tumors.
- MEN2B is a rare genetic mutation that, if not suspected and diagnosed, often results in childhood MTC and early death.
- MEN2B causes MTC, pheochromocytomas, and benign ganglioneuromas.

DISCLOSURE

L.A. Greenberg has no commercial or financial conflicts of interest and no funding sources.

REFERENCES

1. Giusti F, Cianferotti L, Boaretto F, et al. Multiple endocrine neoplasia syndrome type 1: institution, management, and data analysis of a nationwide multicenter patient database. Endocrine 2017;58(2):349–59.
2. Trump D, Farren B, Wooding C, et al. Clinical studies of multiple endocrine neoplasia type 1 (MEN1). QJM 1996;89(9):653–70.
3. Cristina E-V, Alberto F. Management of familial hyperparathyroidism syndromes: MEN1, MEN2, MEN4, HPT-Jaw tumour, Familial isolated hyperparathyroidism, FHH, and neonatal severe hyperparathyroidism. Best Pract Res Clin Endocrinol Metabol 2018;32(6):861–75.
4. Burgess JR, David R, Greenaway TM, et al. Osteoporosis in multiple endocrine neoplasia type 1: severity, clinical significance, relationship to primary hyperparathyroidism, and response to parathyroidectomy. Arch Surg 1999;134(10): 1119–23.
5. Pipeleers-Marichal M, Somers G, Willems G, et al. Gastrinomas in the duodenums of patients with multiple endocrine neoplasia type 1 and the Zollinger-Ellison syndrome. N Engl J Med 1990;322(11):723–7.
6. Thakker RV, Newey PJ, Walls GV, et al. Clinical practice guidelines for multiple endocrine neoplasia type 1 (MEN1). J Clin Endocrinol Metabol 2012;97(9): 2990–3011.
7. McDonnell JE, Gild ML, Clifton-Bligh RJ, et al. Multiple endocrine neoplasia: an update. Int Med J 2019;49(8):954–61.
8. Brandi ML, Gagel RF, Angeli A, et al. Guidelines for diagnosis and therapy of MEN type 1 and type 2. J Clin Endocrinol Metabol 2001;86(12):5658–71.

9. Mathiesen JS, Kroustrup JP, Vestergaard P, et al. Incidence and prevalence of multiple endocrine neoplasia 2A in Denmark 1901-2014: a nationwide study. Clin Epidemiol 2018;10:1479–87.

10. Mathiesen JS, Kroustrup JP, Vestergaard P, et al. Incidence and prevalence of multiple endocrine neoplasia 2B in Denmark: a nationwide study. Endocr Relat Cancer 2017;24(7):L39–42.

11. Modigliani E, Cohen R, Campos J-M, et al. Prognostic factors for survival and for biochemical cure in medullary thyroid carcinoma: results in 899 patients. Clin Endocrinol 1998;48(3):265–73.

12. Schuffenecker I, Ginet N, Goldgar D, et al. Prevalence and parental origin of de novo RET mutations in multiple endocrine neoplasia type 2A and familial medullary thyroid carcinoma. Le Groupe d'Etude des Tumeurs a Calcitonine. Am J Hum Genet 1997;60(1):233–7.

13. Castinetti F, Waguespack SG, Machens A, et al. Natural history, treatment, and long-term follow up of patients with multiple endocrine neoplasia type 2B: an international, multicentre, retrospective study. Lancet Diabetes Endocrinol 2019; 7(3):213–20.

14. Brauckhoff M, Machens A, Lorenz K, et al. Surgical curability of medullary thyroid cancer in multiple endocrine neoplasia 2B: a changing perspective. Ann Surg 2014;259:800–6.

15. Raue F, Frank-Raue K. Genotype-phenotype correlation in multiple endocrine neoplasia type 2. Clinics 2012;67(Suppl 1):69–75.

16. Takahashi M, Ritz J, Cooper GM. Activation of a novel human transforming gene, ret, by DNA rearrangement. Cell 1985;42(2):581–8.

17. Takaya K, Yoshimasa T, Arai H, et al. Expression of the RET proto-oncogene in normal human tissues, pheochromocytomas, and other tumors of neural crest origin. J Mol Med (Berl) 1996;74(10):617–21.

18. Brauckhoff M, Gimm O, Thanh PN, et al. Critical size of residual adrenal tissue and recovery from impaired early postoperative adrenocortical function after subtotal bilateral adrenalectomy. Surgery 2003;134(6):1020–7.

19. Lihara M, Yamashita T, Okamoto T, et al. A Nationwide clinical survey of patients with multiple endocrine neoplasia type 2 and familial medullary thyroid carcinoma in Japan. Jpn J Clin Oncol 1997;27(3):128–34.

20. Wells J, Chi DD, Toshima K, et al. Predictive DNA testing and prophylactic thyroidectomy in patients at risk for multiple endocrine neoplasia type 2A. Ann Surg 1994;220(3):237–50.

21. Scapineli JO, Ceolin L, Puñales MK, et al. MEN 2A related cutaneous lichen amyloidosis: report of three kindred and systematic literature review of clinical, biochemical and molecular characteristics. Fam Cancer 2016;15(4):625–33.

22. Kotecka-Blicharz A, Hasse-Lazar K, Jurecka-Lubieniecka B, et al. Occurrence of phaeochromocytoma tumours in RET mutation carriers — a single-centre study. Endokrynol Pol 2016;67(1):54–8.

23. Martucciello G, Lerone M, Bricco L, et al. Multiple endocrine neoplasias type 2B and RET proto-oncogene. Ital J Pediatr 2012;38(1):9.

24. Shah U, Giubellino A, Pacak K. Pheochromocytoma: implications in tumorigenesis and the actual management. Minerva Endocrinol 2012;37(2):141–56.

25. Haugen BR, Alexander EK, Bible KC, et al. 2015 American Thyroid Association Management Guidelines for adult patients with thyroid nodules and differentiated thyroid cancer: The American Thyroid Association Guidelines task force on thyroid nodules and differentiated thyroid cancer. Thyroid 2016;26(1):1–133.

26. Sippel RS, Kunnimalaiyaan M, Chen H. Current Management of Medullary Thyroid Cancer. Oncol 2008;13(5):539–47.

27. Mathiesen JS, Effraimidis G, Rossing M, et al. Multiple endocrine neoplasia type 2: A review. Semin Cancer Biol 2022;79:163–79.

28. Raue F, Dralle H, Machens A, et al. Long-term survivorship in multiple endocrine neoplasia type 2B diagnosed before and in the new millennium. J Clin Endocrinol Metabol 2018;103(1):235–43.

29. Eng C. The relationship between specific RET proto-oncogene mutations and disease phenotype in multiple endocrine neoplasia type 2. International RET mutation consortium analysis. JAMA, J Am Med Assoc 1996;276(19):1575–9.

30. Gfroerer S, Theilen TM, Fiegel H, et al. Identification of intestinal ganglioneuromatosis leads to early diagnosis of MEN2B: role of rectal biopsy. J Pediatr Surg 2017;52(7):1161–5.

31. Pacak K, Eisenhofer G, Ilias I. Diagnosis of pheochromocytoma with special emphasis on MEN2 syndrome. Hormones (Basel) 2009;8(2):111–6.

32. Gavriilidis P, Camenzuli C, Paspala A, et al. Posterior Retroperitoneoscopic versus laparoscopic transperitoneal adrenalectomy: a systematic review by an updated meta-analysis. World J Surg 2021;45(1):168–79.

Endocrine Emergencies

Abdul Waheed, MD, MS PHS, CPE[a],*, Shehar Bano Awais, MD[b],
Sukhjeet Kamboj, MD[b], Hussain Mahmud, MD[c]

KEYWORDS

- Endocrine emergencies • Thyrotoxicosis • Myxedema coma • Addisonian crisis
- Ketoacidosis • Pituitary • Hypercalcemia • Hypocalcemia

KEY POINTS

- Endocrine emergencies span a range of conditions involving glands including the thyroid, parathyroid, pituitary, pancreas, and adrenal glands, characterized by either an excess or deficiency of hormone levels.
- Clinical presentation may be nonspecific, which may delay diagnosis. However, it is crucial to begin treatment without delay before a diagnosis is made.
- Management involves a team approach. Therefore, enhanced awareness among health care professionals for swift intervention in these critical scenarios can decrease mortality rates.

THYROID EMERGENCIES: THYROID STORM AND MYEDEMA COMA
Thyroid Storm or Acute Thyrotoxicosis

Definitions
Hyperthyroidism. Elevated levels of thyroid hormones in the blood may occur as the result of increased synthesis and release of thyroid hormones from the thyroid gland.[1]

Thyrotoxicosis. Clinical manifestations and symptoms resulting from increased thyroid hormones in the blood. Severity may range from overt thyrotoxicosis to more severe thyroid storm.[2]

Thyroid storm. Acute, life-threatening condition characterized by an exaggerated manifestation of thyrotoxic state resulting in end-organ damage or decompensation.[2]

---

[a] Department of Family Medicine, Dignity Health Medical Group, Creighton University School of Medicine, Phoenix, AZ, USA; [b] WellSpan Good Samaritan Hospital Family Medicine Residency Program, PO Box 1520, Lebanon, PA 17042, USA; [c] Department of Medicine, Endocrinology Division, UPMC Center for Endocrinology & Metabolism, University of Pittsburgh Medical College, 3601 5th Avenue, Falk Suite 3B, Pittsburgh, PA 15213, USA
* Corresponding author. Department of Family Medicine, Dignity Health Medical Group, Suite 2021, Gilbert, AZ 85297.
E-mail address: Abdul.waheed@commonspirit.org
Twitter: @WaheedMD123 (A.W.); @Sheharbanoawais (S.B.A.)

Prim Care Clin Office Pract 51 (2024) 495–510
https://doi.org/10.1016/j.pop.2024.04.006
primarycare.theclinics.com
0095-4543/24/© 2024 Elsevier Inc. All rights reserved.

Epidemiology

In the United States, the incidence of thyroid storm is 0.57 to 0.76 per 100,000 persons per year, with a higher incidence in hospitalized patients (4.8–5.6/100,000). The average age is 42 to 43 years, and the male:female ratio is 1:3.[3]

Causes and triggers

There are many factors including infection, trauma, and abrupt discontinuation of thioamide (methimazole, carbimazole, propylthiouracil) therapy that could potentially trigger the development of thyroid storm. These are summarized in **Table 1**.[4,5] Underlying Graves' disease is noteworthy as it may increase the risk of acute thyroid storm; however, 24% to 43% of the cases of thyroid storm have no identifiable trigger.

Presentation

The clinical presentation during thyroid storm is often variable and patients may present with nonspecific findings. **Fig. 1** shows features commonly present at the time of diagnosis. Most findings are due to the amplified effects of the thyroid hormone causing increased oxygen consumption and increased activity of sympathetic nervous system.

Evaluation and diagnosis

The diagnostic laboratories and imaging tests are summarized in **Table 2**. The diagnosis of thyroid storm must be made based on clinical findings. Moreover, laboratory tests to determine thyroid function may not be significantly different from other thyrotoxic states and therefore inconclusive when trying to diagnose thyroid storm. Fever (>39 C or 102°F) is the most common sign, and thyroid storm should be highly considered in a patient presenting with fever and known thyroid disease.[5] Diagnostic criteria such as the Burch–Wartofsky point scale may assist in diagnosis; however, it should not be used in isolation as a high score lacks specificity to thyroid storm and can be seen in other conditions such as sepsis.[6]

Management

Thyroid storm is a life-threatening condition with high mortality if left untreated; therefore, effective treatment must be initiated prior to test results. Initial management involves admission to the intensive care unit (ICU), decreasing body temperature using antipyretics, and volume resuscitation using isotonic intravenous (IV) fluids to account for fluid loss secondary to vomiting or diarrhea.[7] Medical therapy includes beta-blockers, antithyroid hormone therapy, inorganic iodide, and corticosteroid

Table 1 Identified triggers of thyroid storm[4]	
Thyroid disease	Graves' disease, toxic multinodular goiter
Infection:	Any bacterial or viral infection, postviral thyroiditis, and suppurative thyroiditis
Pregnancy related	Pregnancy, labor, postpartum thyroiditis, struma ovarii, and molar pregnancy
Stress:	Trauma, burns, MI, PE, stroke, DKA, and intense exercise
Malignancy:	Metastatic or benign thyroid cancer resulting in goiter
Iatrogenic	Discontinuation of antithyroid medications, overdose of thyroid hormone, amiodarone, thyroid surgery
Toxins:	Certain drugs such as salicylates, organophosphates

Abbreviations: DKA, diabetes ketoacidosis; MI, myocardial infarction; PE, pulmonary embolism.

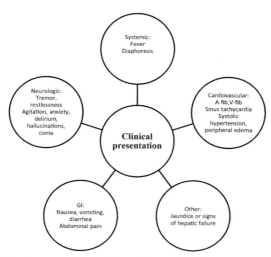

Fig. 1. Common clinical presentation of thyroid storm.[2,4,5]

therapy. Since infection is one of the most common precipitating factors, the American Thyroid Association (ATA) recommends starting an empiric broad-spectrum antibiotic. Medical therapy is aimed at the following mechanisms[8]:

1. To control an increased adrenergic tone, beta-blockers with a short half-life, for example, propranolol and esmolol are preferred. However, the use of beta-blockers should be avoided in acute decompensated heart failure with systolic dysfunction.
2. To reduce thyroid hormone synthesis and release, the use of thioamides should be considered. Propylthiouracil (PTU) is preferred over methimazole due to its impact on T4 to T3 conversion. Inorganic iodine solution should only be administered after thioamide initiation.

Table 2
Common laboratories and imaging to obtain when suspecting thyroid storm[5,6]

Laboratory/Imaging	Reasoning
CBC, inflammatory markers, urinalysis, chest X-ray (CXR)	To rule out infection, anemia, and assess for heart failure
Thyroid-stimulating hormone (TSH), T3, and free T4	To evaluate thyroid function. May be inconclusive
Complete metabolic profile, CK	To check for renal and liver function. Electrolyte disturbances may trigger thyroid storm
EKG	Arrhythmias such as atrial fibrillation, common in 10%–30% cases of thyroid storm
Urine drug screen	Certain toxins may trigger thyroid storm
Beta-human chorionic gonadotropin	Pregnancy and certain conditions during pregnancy may precipitate disease
Computed tomography (CT) head	To rule out neurologic causes (such as pituitary adenoma)

Abbreviations: CBC, complete blood count; CK, creatinine kinase; EKG, electrocardiogram.

3. To block peripheral conversion of T4 to T3, one should use corticosteroids. PTU and beta-blockers also help with blocking the peripheral conversion of T4 to T3.
4. Reduce enterohepatic recycling of thyroid hormone by using bile acid sequestrants (eg, cholestyramine).

Effective management can be summarized with the mnemonic "B.A.S.I.C.":

B: B-adrenergic blockers, broad-spectrum antibiotics
A: Antithyroid hormone therapy
S: Sequestrants (bile acid sequestrants)
I: Inorganic iodide, ICU admission, IV fluids
C: Corticosteroid therapy

Myxedema Coma

Introduction

Myxedema coma is defined as decompensated hypothyroidism leading to multiorgan failure.[9] The exact incidence is unknown; however, studies show it ranges from 0.22 to 1.08 cases per million patients per year. Women aged above 60 years and those with a history of hypothyroidism are most affected.[10] "Myxedema coma" is often considered as a misnomer as the prime manifestation of the disease is deterioration of mental status, and most patients neither present with nonpitting edema (myxedema) nor coma.

Among these causes, failure to continue thyroid replacement therapy and infections are the most common risk factors that lead to the development of myxedema coma.[11,12] **Table 3** lists common precipitating factors of myxedema coma.

Clinical presentation

The clinical presentation and findings can be accounted for by the loss of thermogenesis, reduced metabolism, depression of the central respiratory system, and decreased gluconeogenesis.[13] The neurologic change may present as lethargy and obtundation or an activated state known as "myxedema madness."[14] **Fig. 2** summarizes typical features at presentation while **Table 3** indicates common precipitating factors.

Diagnosis

If a patient with known hypothyroidism presents with depressed mental status and hypothermia in the setting of a precipitating event, myxedema coma should be highly considered.[15] Diagnostic criteria are available but have not been widely assessed on different patient populations.[16] Recommended laboratory work and imaging include

Table 3 Common precipitating factors of myxedema coma[11,12]	
Medications	Discontinuation or inability to start thyroid medications in a patient with known hypothyroidism or the use of sedatives, narcotics, and anesthetics
Infections	Most commonly pneumonia or urosepsis
Cardiovascular	Congestive heart failure
Obstetric	Labor
Neurologic	Cerebrovascular events
Environment	Low temperature
Trauma	Fractures, injury

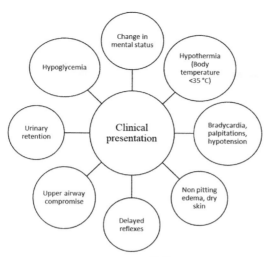

Fig. 2. Clinical presentation of myxedema coma.[13,14]

- CBC, inflammatory markers, urinalysis: to evaluate for infectious processes
- Arterial blood gases: to diagnose respiratory acidosis, hypercapnia, and hypoxia
- TSH, T4, T3: to evaluate thyroid function (most patients have elevated TSH and low T4)
- CK: to rule out rhabdomyolysis resulting from urinary retention
- Complete metabolic profile: electrolyte abnormalities specifically hyponatremia
- EKG: evaluate for arrhythmias, heart block, and torsades de point
- Echocardiogram and CXR: for pleural effusion or cardiomegaly
- MRI pituitary: to look for causes of secondary hypothyroidism (pituitary macroadenoma, empty sella)

Management

It is essential to initiate lifesaving treatment prior to waiting for laboratory results as that may delay the treatment course. An outline of general management of myxedema coma is shown in **Fig. 3**. Management includes admitting the patient to the ICU for continued monitoring and beginning prompt thyroid replacement therapy. A combination of parenteral levothyroxine and liothyronine is recommended.[17,18] Typically, one can start with a load of 200 to 400 mg of levothyroxine IV, followed by 50 to 100 mg IV daily. Liothyronine is administered concomitantly 5 to 20 mcg as loading dose

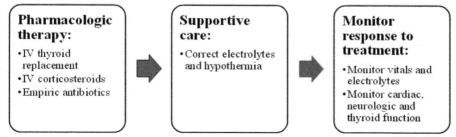

Fig. 3. Outline of the management of myxedema coma.[17–19]

followed by 2.5 to 10 mcg IV every 8 hours. The ATA recommends that after the initial loading doses, up titration in response to symptoms and switch to oral as soon as patient is able to tolerate oral.[18]

In addition to thyroid replacement, electrolyte abnormalities such as hyponatremia should be corrected with IV normal saline infusion. Passive rewarming methods including blankets should be to raise body temperature and prevent life-threatening hypothermia. Active rewarming methods using heated blankets are not recommended and may result in worsening hypotension due to peripheral dilation. Infections such as pneumonia and urosepsis are a precipitating factor for myxedema coma; therefore, empiric antibiotics should be started early. Moreover, IV corticosteroid therapy (hydrocortisone 100 mg then 50 mg q6hours) should be initiated until coexisting adrenal insufficiency is ruled out. Cardiac function, urinary output, neurologic function, vitals, and thyroid function should be closely monitored. Eventually, patients can be transitioned to oral thyroid replacement therapy based on clinical improvement.[19]

PARATHYROID EMERGENCIES: HYPERCALCEMIC CRISIS AND HYPOCALCEMIC CRISIS
Hypercalcemic Crisis

Epidemiology and pathophysiology
Hypercalcemic crisis is an uncommon condition in which patients develop severe hypercalcemia with signs and symptoms of multiorgan dysfunction. Primary hyperparathyroidism, is one of the most common causes of hypercalcemic crisis.[20]

Presentation
Common signs and symptoms of hypercalcemia crisis may be general (generalized weakness and malaise) musculoskeletal (bone pain, fractures, and muscle weakness), nephrogenic (anuria, oliguria, nocturia, nephrolithiasis, and acute renal failure), or gastrointestinal (abdominal pain, constipation, and vomiting).[21] Patients may also present with complications of hypercalcemia including pancreatitis, nephrolithiasis, and cardiac arrhythmias.

Diagnosis and workup
Diagnostic workup for hypercalcemia can be extensive. **Table 4** lists common laboratory tests and imaging procedures that may be done to determine the etiology of hypercalcemic crisis and to monitor the resulting end-organ dysfunction.

Hypoalbuminemia may alter calcium levels in blood; therefore, it is important to calculate corrected blood calcium using the following formula.
Corrected calcium = serum calcium + 0.8 × (4 − serum albumin).[22]

An exact cutoff to diagnose hypercalcemic crisis has not been decided; however, the calculated albumin-corrected blood calcium level in hypercalcemic crisis is usually greater than 14 mg/dL. [23]

Management
The mortality rate due to parathyroid crisis was previously reported to be as high as 66%; however, it has decreased over time due to early recognition and improved treatment.[24] If calcium level persistently remains critically elevated, the organs most affected and prone to decompensation are the brain and kidneys, potentially resulting in irreversible coma or renal failure.[25]

Therefore, early recognition of the disease and initiation of treatment is important. Medications such as digoxin and hydrochlorothiazide should be avoided as they increase mortality.[20] Preoperative supportive measures that have demonstrated efficacy in improving the clinical condition of patients include[25,26]

Table 4
Common workup in suspected hypercalcemic crisis[6]

Laboratory Tests	Rationale
Calcium, ionized calcium, and albumin	To confirm hypercalcemia and calculate corrected calcium
Parathyroid hormone (PTH)	To differentiate between PTH-mediated and non-PTH-mediated etiologies
25-hydroxyvitamin D	To evaluate the impact of vitamin D deficiency-mediated secondary hyperparathyroidism on PTH level
Complete metabolic profile	Elevated BUN and creatinine are often seen in hypercalcemia. To evaluate liver function, kidney function, and to plan electrolyte repletion
Urine studies (including urine protein) PTHrP, 1,25-dihydroxyvitamin D and SPEP/UPEP	To evaluate non-PTH-mediated hypercalcemia etiologies
Imaging	
EKG	To evaluate for arrhythmias
Parathyroid sestamibi scan and neck ultrasound	Performed for localization of enlarged parathyroid glands, once primary hyperparathyroidism has been confirmed biochemically

Abbreviations: PTHrP, parathyroid hormone related peptide; SPEP, serum protein electrophoresis; UPEP, urine protein electrophoresis.

1. Rehydration: Aggressive IV rehydration with isotonic saline to counteract hypercalcemia-driven osmotic diuresis and argenine vassopressin (AVP) resistance.
2. Calcium lowering therapy: IV calcitonin and IV infusion of bisphosphonates such as pamidronate and zoledronic acid. Denosumab is the preferred agent among patients with severe acute kidney injury (AKI).
3. Loop diuretics: to promote calciuresis, only if patient appears to have fluid overload.
   Hypercalcemic crisis secondary to hyperparathyroidism is considered a surgical emergency and surgical parathyroidectomy within 24 to 72 hours remains the definitive treatment option.[21] Therefore, ectopic release of parathyroid hormone must be ruled out, and the diagnosis must be established early to plan for necessary surgical treatment.

Hypocalcemic Crisis

Epidemiology and etiology
Hypoparathyroidism is an uncommon condition, with an estimated incidence of 37 per 100,000 person-years in the United States and can result in potentially life-threatening hypocalcemia.[27] Anterior neck surgery accounts for about 75% of cases of hypoparathyroidism, but it can also be due to autoimmune conditions, radiation, and metastatic disease.[28]

Clinical Presentation

Table 5 lists signs and symptoms of acute hypocalcemia.[29]

Diagnosis
Laboratory testing aims to assess parathyroid function and exclude other electrolyte abnormalities (hypomagnesemia) or disorders that might manifest with comparable

Table 5
Common clinical presentation of acute hypocalcemia

Neuromuscular excitability	Chvostek's sign, Trousseau's sign, paresthesias, tetany, seizures (focal, generalized), muscle cramps and weakness, dystonic spasms, laryngospasm, and bronchospasm
Mental status	Confusion, disorientation, psychosis, personality changes, irritability, impaired intellectual ability, and parkinsonism
Cardiac	Palpitations, signs of congestive heart failure (dyspnea and edema)
Smooth muscle involvement	Dysphagia, abdominal pain, biliary colic, dyspnea, and wheezing

clinical signs. Initial laboratory analysis involves assessing serum levels of calcium, phosphate, magnesium, intact PTH, 25-hydroxyvitamin D, and 1,25-dihydroxyvitamin D alongside measuring albumin level to calculate corrected serum calcium.[29] **Table 6** lists recommended investigations to aid in the diagnosis of hypocalcemia.

Treatment

Acute hypocalcemia is considered an emergency, requiring immediate attention. If not addressed promptly, acute hypocalcemia has the potential to rapidly advance, resulting in diverse neurologic and cardiac complications that can ultimately lead to death. Complications include seizures, status epilepticus, coma, or life-threatening cardiac arrhythmias.[30]

The typical threshold for initiating acute management is a calcium level of 1.9 mmol/L (7.5 mg/dL)[30]; however, the decision to administer acute therapy is also guided by symptoms. Emergent treatment of hypocalcemia with IV calcium gluconate is preferred, as IV calcium chloride often causes local irritation. The infusion should be continued until the patient is asymptomatic or calcium level returns to normal. In patients with end-stage renal failure or those on dialysis, large-volume calcium infusions should be avoided. Potential hazards of IV calcium administration, although uncommon, include local thrombophlebitis, cardiotoxicity, hypotension, calcium taste, flushing.[31]

Prevention

Some protocols advocate administering calcium and calcitriol postoperatively after thyroid surgery, regardless of serum calcium levels, to reduce the risk of developing hypocalcemia. Additionally, perioperative PTH concentration, preoperative vitamin

Table 6
Common workup for suspected acute hypocalcemia crisis[29]

Laboratory Tests	Rationale
Serum total calcium, ionized calcium	Assess extent of hypocalcemia
Phosphate	Assess for hypophosphatemia
PTH	Assess for primary hypoparathyroidism
Magnesium	Hypomagnesemia may lead to impaired release of PTH
Vitamin D levels	Low vitamin D levels result in low calcium absorption
Electrocardiogram	Hypocalcemia leads to prolonged Q wave to T wave (QT) and arrhythmias
Neck ultrasound	Investigate structural abnormalities of parathyroid gland
Urine calcium	To distinguish between renal and nonrenal etiology

D levels, and early postoperative changes in calcium levels serve as useful biochemical predictors of postthyroidectomy hypocalcemia.[32]

ADRENAL EMERGENCIES: ADRENAL CRISIS AND PHEOCHROMOCYTOMA
Adrenal Crisis/Addisonian Crisis

Introduction
An adrenal crisis is a critical endocrine emergency that arises from the insufficient production of the adrenal hormone cortisol, a primary glucocorticoid. This life-threatening condition can stem from either primary adrenal insufficiency, characterized by the impaired function of the adrenal gland itself, or secondary adrenal insufficiency, where the regulation of adrenal cortisol production by the pituitary is compromised.

In adults, an adrenal crisis is characterized by a sudden decline in health marked by either absolute hypotension (systolic blood pressure <100 mm Hg) or relative hypotension (systolic blood pressure ≥20 mm Hg lower than usual). This condition is typically associated with symptoms that show marked improvement within 1 to 2 hours after the administration of parenteral glucocorticoids.[33] Every year, around 6% to 8% of individuals with adrenal insufficiency experience an episode of adrenal crisis. Literature indicates a prevalence of adrenal crisis ranging from 5.2 to 8.3 per 100 patient years.[34]

Causes and triggers
A number of factors have been implicated in precipitating Addisonian or adrenal crisis. **Table 7** lists common precipitating factors leading to adrenal crisis.[33]

Clinical presentation
Patients may present with variable symptoms including abdominal pain, anorexia, nausea, vomiting, fatigue, postural dizziness, and impaired consciousness or coma.[35]

Diagnosis
Common laboratory findings include hyponatremia, hyperkalemia, hypercalcemia, hypoglycemia, neutropenia, eosinophilia, lymphocytosis, and normocytic anemia.[33]

If there is suspicion of an adrenal crisis, it is advisable to draw a blood sample promptly for serum cortisol and adrenocorticotropic hormone (ACTH); however, treatment should commence without waiting for assay results.[36] ACTH stimulation test, a diagnostic tool employed under stable conditions (involving the measurement of serum cortisol at baseline, 30 and 60 minutes after an IV injection of ACTH 250 µg), is of limited utility in emergency situations and could unnecessarily prolong the initiation of treatment.[37]

Treatment
Treatment should be initiated as soon as adrenal crisis is suspected as commencing lifesaving hydrocortisone treatment poses no adverse consequences. Treatment is aimed at the following[38]:

1. Glucocorticoid replacement: prompt administration of IV hydrocortisone 50 to 100 mg. This can be followed by hydrocortisone 50 mg IV every 6 hours or a continuous infusion.
2. Rapid rehydration: Rehydration involves a rapid IV infusion of 1000 mL of isotonic saline.
3. Treating the precipitating event: For example, treatment with antibiotics may be necessary in the setting of infection.

Following the successful management of an adrenal crisis, the hydrocortisone doses should be gradually tapered. An assessment for potential preventable triggers should be conducted, and the patient should be educated about preventive strategies.[36]

Table 7 Common triggers precipitating adrenal crisis[33]		
Primary adrenal insufficiency	Stress induced	Infections, Trauma, surgery, and psychological stress
	Ischemia	Due to major blood loss
	Hemorrhage	Waterhouse–Friderichsen disease (secondary to *Neisseria meningitidis* infection), peripartum, disseminated intravascular coagulation (DIC), and anticoagulant use
	Iatrogenic	Nonadherence to glucocorticoid replacement therapy
Secondary adrenal insufficiency	Hypothalamic-pituitary related	Pituitary tumor, Sheehan's syndrome, and pituitary apoplexy Chronic glucocorticoid use

Pheochromocytoma Crisis

Introduction

Pheochromocytoma is a rare tumor that results in excess production of catecholamines and can lead to pheochromocytoma crisis, which can be classified as type A and type B. Type A crisis includes hemodynamic instability and evidence of end-organ dysfunction of least one-organ system. Type A (limited crisis) may progress to type B (extensive crisis and shock), which has a higher mortality rate, and is characterized by sustained hypotension and multiorgan dysfunction.[39]

Symptoms

Pheochromocytoma crisis typically presents with hypertensive emergency. Other conditions and complications associated with pheochromocytoma crisis include stroke, arrhythmias, acute coronary syndrome, pulmonary edema, respiratory failure, seizure, multiorgan failure, and death.[39]

Evaluation

Acute evaluation varies based on symptomatology, but typically includes a CBC, complete metabolic profile (CMP), TSH, toxicology, electrocardiogram, CXR, and abdominal CT.[39]

Treatment

Alpha blockade hypertensive emergency treatment is used to treat hypertension, and IV phentolamine is commonly recommended.[39] Other treatments vary based on the individual case and presentation and may include the need for ventilatory support.

PANCREATIC ENDOCRINE EMERGENCIES: DIABETIC KETOACIDOSIS
Part 1: Diabetic Ketoacidosis

Introduction

DKA is an acute complication of diabetes mellitus that carries a high-risk of mortality if not treated appropriately. It stands as the primary cause of mortality in individuals aged under 24 years with diabetes, primarily attributed to cerebral edema in many cases.[40] In approximately 25% to 40% of patients with type 1 diabetes, DKA may manifest as the initial presentation.[41] Initially believed to be exclusive to individuals with type 1 diabetes, DKA has also been identified in patients with type 2 diabetes under specific conditions.

Pathophysiology
The primary triggers in most cases are the onset of new diabetes, infection, or noncompliance with prescribed treatment.[42] Additional precipitating factors include alcohol abuse, trauma, pulmonary embolism, and myocardial infarction.[43]

Signs and symptoms
Typical manifestations of DKA include[42]

1. General symptoms: reduced urine output, dry mouth, poor capillary refill, and decreased sweating
2. Respiratory: dyspnea, fruity smell in breath, and Kussmaul (labored, deep, and rapid breathing)
3. Gastrointestinal: vomiting, abdominal pain and tenderness, anorexia, and nausea
4. Neurologic: Altered mental status, general drowsiness, and focal neurologic deficits (may occur in severe cases as a sign of cerebral edema)

Diagnosis
The diagnostic criteria for DKA as per the guidelines of the American Diabetes Association is outlined in **Table 8**.

In addition to evaluating blood glucose levels, blood pH, serum bicarbonate, ketones, and calculated anion gap, further laboratory investigations are typically conducted to assess the underlying cause and potential complications. A sepsis workup is carried out assessing lactate levels, complete blood count (which may reveal leukocytosis), and complete metabolic profile (particularly assessing electrolyte imbalances such as hypokalemia and hyponatremia). Additionally, a comprehensive investigation includes urinalysis, blood culture, urine culture, and a chest radiograph to diagnose potential infections. Osmotic diuresis and natriuresis result in a general depletion of electrolytes. Consequently, an EKG is conducted to exclude arrhythmias that may arise as a secondary effect of electrolyte imbalances.

Management
Failure to treat DKA can lead to severe complications that may be fatal, including arrhythmias, cerebral edema, respiratory failure, and rhabdomyolysis. Hence, swift recognition of the disease and prompt initiation of treatment are imperative.

The therapeutic objectives for individuals experiencing hyperglycemic crises involve the following[41]:

Table 8
Diagnostic criteria for diabetic ketoacidosis as per American Diabetes Association guidelines[43,44]

	Mild	Moderate	Severe
Serum pH	7.25–7.30	7.00 to <7.24	<7.00
Blood glucose	>250	>250	>250
Serum bicarbonate (mEq/L)	15–18	10 to <15	<10
Urine and serum ketones	Positive	Positive	Positive
Anion gap	10	>12	>12
Mental status	Alert	Alert/drowsy	Stupor/coma

1. Administering IV fluids to improve tissue perfusion: **Fig. 4** for a concise flowchart on IV rehydration.
2. Initiating insulin therapy to lower serum glucose: Start with a bolus of IV regular insulin 0.1 U/kg followed by 0.1 U/kg/h continuous infusion. The insulin infusion dose can be doubled if serum glucose does not fall by 50 to 70 mg/dL in the first hour of treatment. Adjust and reduce the insulin infusion to 0.05 to 0.1 U/kg/h once serum glucose reaches 300 mg/dL.
3. Repletion of potassium: Replete potassium before initiating insulin infusion if serum levels are below 3.3 mEq/L. For levels between 3.3 and 5.3 mEq, add 20 to 30 mEq of potassium to each liter of fluid administered. Monitor serum potassium every 2 hours if levels exceed 5.3.
4. Assessing the need for bicarbonate: Administer bicarbonate if serum pH is below 6.9; otherwise, no intervention is needed.
5. Promptly identifying and treating precipitating causes.

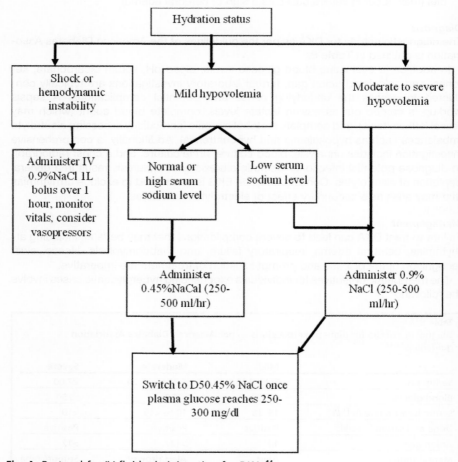

Fig. 4. Protocol for IV fluid administration for DKA.[41]

PITUITARY EMERGENCIES: PITUITARY APOPLEXY
Pituitary Apoplexy

Epidemiology
Pituitary apoplexy is a rare clinical syndrome where there is hemorrhage or infarct of the pituitary gland. It occurs in 2% to 12% of pituitary adenomas, with a higher prevalence among nonfunctioning macroadenomas.[45] If not identified and addressed promptly, pituitary apoplexy can pose a life-threatening risk with overall mortality rates between 1.6% and 1.9%.[46] Factors contributing to pituitary apoplexy may include surgical procedures resulting in reduced blood flow, stimulation applied to the pituitary gland, and the use of anticoagulant medications in patients.

Clinical presentation
Pituitary apoplexy commonly presents with a primary symptom of headache, often accompanied by visual field impairment or ocular palsies, with bitemporal hemianopsia being the most prevalent. They can present with cognitive changes and may manifest symptoms of meningeal irritation, such as photophobia, nausea, and vomiting.[47] Furthermore, multiple acute endocrine insufficiencies including deficiencies in anterior pituitary hormones like ACTH and TSH may occur simultaneously, leading to symptoms of acute adrenal and thyroid insufficiency.

Diagnosis
MRI is the preferred radiological investigation and has been proven effective in confirming the diagnosis of pituitary apoplexy.[47]

Treatment
In the management of pituitary apoplexy, providers should prioritize hemodynamic stability. Maintaining electrolyte balance, replacement of deficient hormone, and making referrals to endocrine and neurosurgery specialists are also crucial steps. Since corticotropic deficiency is prevalent in most patients, IV corticosteroids (IV hydrocortisone) should be promptly administered upon confirming the diagnosis.[48]

The decision to pursue conservative or surgical management should be made by a multidisciplinary team of experts. Surgery, often utilizing a trans-sphenoidal approach, has demonstrated the highest efficacy in addressing pituitary apoplexy.[49]

Prognosis
Surgical decompression typically leads to improvement in altered consciousness, and visual field, especially when they were normal before the acute episode. Ophthalmoplegia usually resolves, but the process may take several weeks. Endocrine function often remains mildly altered even after treatment; therefore, long-term follow-up, both endocrine assessment and imaging, is necessary.[45]

DISCLOSURE

The authors have nothing to disclose.

REFERENCES

1. De Leo S, Lee SY, Braverman LE. Hyperthyroidism. Lancet 2016;388(10047): 906–18.
2. Chiha M, Samarasinghe S, Kabaker AS. Thyroid storm. J Intensive Care Med 2013;30(3):131–40.
3. Galindo RJ, Hurtado CR, Pasquel FJ, et al. National trends in incidence, mortality, and clinical outcomes of patients hospitalized for thyrotoxicosis with and without

thyroid storm in the United States, 2004–2013. Thyroid 2019;29(1):36–43. https://doi.org/10.1089/THY.2018.0275. Available at: https://home.liebertpub.com/thy.

7. Farooqi S, Raj S, Koyfman A, et al. High risk and low prevalence diseases: Thyroid storm. Am J Emerg Med 2023;69:127–35.

4. Burch HB, Wartofsky L. Life-threatening thyrotoxicosis: thyroid storm. Endocrinol Metab Clin N Am 1993;22(2):263–77.

6. Pearce EN. Diagnosis and management of thyrotoxicosis. BMJ 2006;332(7554): 1369.

5. Carroll R, Matfin G. Endocrine and metabolic emergencies: thyroid storm. Ther Adv Endocrinol Metab 2010;1(3):139.

8. De Almeida R, McCalmon S, Cabandugama PK. Clinical review and update on the management of thyroid storm. Mo Med 2022;119(4):366. Available at: http://pmc/articles/PMC9462913/. [Accessed 6 February 2024].

9. DeSanctis V, Soliman A, Daar S, et al. Myxedema coma in children and adolescents: A rare endocrine emergency - Personal experience and review of literature. Acta Bio Medica Atenei Parm 2021;92(5):2021481.

10. Ono Y, Ono S, Yasunaga H, et al. Clinical characteristics and outcomes of myxedema coma: Analysis of a national inpatient database in Japan. J Epidemiol 2017;27(3):117–22.

11. Wall CR. Myxedema coma: diagnosis and treatment. Am Fam Physician 2000; 62(11):2485–90. Available at: https://www.aafp.org/pubs/afp/issues/2000/1201/p2485.html. [Accessed 22 November 2023].

12. Papi G, Corsello SM, Pontecorvi A. Clinical concepts on thyroid emergencies. Front Endocrinol 2014;5(JUL):98169.

13. Mathew V, Misgar RA, Ghosh S, et al. Myxedema coma: a new look into an old crisis. J Thyroid Res 2011;2011. https://doi.org/10.4061/2011/493462.

14. Mavroson MM, Patel N, Akker E. Myxedema psychosis in a patient with undiagnosed hashimoto thyroiditis. J Am Osteopath Assoc 2017;117(1):50–4.

15. Wiersinga WM. Myxedema and coma (severe hypothyroidism). Endotext; 2018. Available at: https://www.ncbi.nlm.nih.gov/books/NBK279007/. [Accessed 22 November 2023].

16. Savarino A, Boelaert JR, Cassone A, et al. Effects of chloroquine on viral infections: An old drug against today's diseases? Lancet Infect Dis 2003;3(11):722–7.

17. Elghawy O, Hafey AC, McCartney CR, et al. Successful treatment of myxedema coma using levothyroxine and liothyronine in the setting of adrenal crisis and severe cardiogenic shock in a patient with apparent primary empty sella. J Clin Transl Endocrinol Case Reports 2021;22:100095.

18. Jonklaas J, Bianco AC, Bauer AJ, et al. Guidelines for the treatment of hypothyroidism: prepared by the american thyroid association task force on thyroid hormone replacement. Thyroid 2014;24(12):1670–751.

19. Hampton J. Thyroid gland disorder emergencies: thyroid storm and myxedema coma. AACN Adv Crit Care 2013;24(3):325–32.

20. Wermers RA, Khosla S, Atkinson EJ, et al. Incidence of primary hyperparathyroidism in Rochester, Minnesota, 1993-2001: an update on the changing epidemiology of the disease. J Bone Miner Res 2006;21(1):171–7.

25. ZIEGLER R. Hypercalcemic crisis. J Am Soc Nephrol 2001;12(suppl_1):S3–9.

21. Ahmad S, Kuraganti G, Steenkamp D. Hypercalcemic crisis: a clinical review. Am J Med 2015;128(3):239–45.

22. Payne RB, Little AJ, Williams RB, et al. Interpretation of serum calcium in patients with abnormal serum proteins. Br Med J 1973;4(5893):643.

23. Omotosho YB, Zahra F. Resistant hypercalcemia. StatPearls 2023. Available at: https://www.ncbi.nlm.nih.gov/books/NBK572109/. [Accessed 27 November 2023].

24. Kutner FR, Morton JH. Parathyroid crisis. Arch Surg 1965;91(1):71–6.

26. Phitayakorn R, McHenry CR. Hyperparathyroid crisis: use of bisphosphonates as a bridge to parathyroidectomy. J Am Coll Surg 2008;206(6):1106–15.

27. Clarke BL, Brown EM, Collins MT, et al. Epidemiology and diagnosis of hypoparathyroidism. J Clin Endocrinol Metab 2016;101(6):2284–99.

28. Bilezikian JP, Khan A, Potts JT, et al. Hypoparathyroidism in the adult: Epidemiology, diagnosis, pathophysiology, target-organ involvement, treatment, and challenges for future research. J Bone Miner Res 2011;26(10):2317–37.

29. Schafer AL, Shoback DM. Hypocalcemia: diagnosis and treatment. Endotext; 2015. Available at: http://europepmc.org/books/NBK279022. [Accessed 28 November 2023].

30. Duval M, Bach-Ngohou K, Masson D, et al. Is severe hypocalcemia immediately life threatening? Endocr Connect 2018;7(10):1067.

31. Turner J, Gittoes N, Selby P, et al. Society for endocrinology endocrine emergency guidance: Emergencymanagement of acute hypocalcaemia in adult patients. Endocr Connect 2016;5(5):G7.

32. Edafe O, Antakia R, Laskar N, et al. Systematic review and meta-analysis of predictors of post-thyroidectomy hypocalcaemia. Br J Surg 2014;101(4):307–20.

33. Elshimy G, Chippa V, Kaur J, et al. Adrenal crisis. StatPearls 2023. Available at: https://www.ncbi.nlm.nih.gov/books/NBK499968/. [Accessed 28 November 2023].

34. Smans LCCJ, Van Der Valk ES, Hermus ARMM, et al. Incidence of adrenal crisis in patients with adrenal insufficiency. Clin Endocrinol (Oxf) 2016;84(1):17–22.

35. Puar THK, Stikkelbroeck NMML, Smans LCCJ, et al. Adrenal crisis: still a deadly event in the 21st century. Am J Med 2016;129(3):339, e1-e9.

36. Dineen R, Thompson CJ, Sherlock M. Adrenal crisis: prevention and management in adult patients. Ther Adv Endocrinol Metab 2019;10. https://doi.org/10.1177/2042018819848218/ASSET/IMAGES/LARGE/10.1177_2042018819848218-FIG1.JPEG.

37. Venkatesh B, Cohen J, Cooper M. Ten false beliefs about cortisol in critically ill patients. Intensive Care Med 2015;41(10):1817–9.

38. Arlt W. Society for Endocrinology Clinical Committee. Emergency management of acute adrenal insufficiency (adrenal crisis) in adult patients. Endocr Connect 2016. https://doi.org/10.1530/EC-16-0054.

39. Bartikoski SR, Reschke DJ. Pheochromocytoma crisis in the emergency department. Cureus 2021 Mar 3;13(3):e13683.

40. J W, N G, MA S, et al. Diabetic ketoacidosis in infants, children, and adolescents: A consensus statement from the American Diabetes Association. Diabetes Care 2006;29(5):1150–9.

41. Calimag APP, Chlebek S, Lerma EV, et al. Diabetic ketoacidosis. Disease-a-Month 2023;69(3):101418.

42. Shahid W, Khan F, Makda A, et al. Diabetic ketoacidosis: clinical characteristics and precipitating factors. Cureus 2020;12(10):e10792.

43. Eledrisi MS, Alshanti MS, Shah MF, et al. Overview of the Diagnosis and Management of Diabetic Ketoacidosis. Am J Med Sci 2006;331(5):243–51.

44. Kitabchi AE, Umpierrez GE, Miles JM, et al. Hyperglycemic crises in adult patients with diabetes. Diabetes Care 2009;32(7):1335–43.

45. Briet C, Salenave S, Bonneville JF, et al. Pituitary Apoplexy. Endocr Rev 2015; 36(6):622–45.

46. Rock J, Asmaro KP. Pituitary Apoplexy. Acute Care Neurosurg by Case Manag Pearls Pitfalls 2023;205–14. https://doi.org/10.1007/978-3-030-99512-6_16.

47. Sibal L, Ball SG, Connolly V, et al. Pituitary apoplexy: a review of clinical presentation, management and outcome in 45 cases. Pituitary 2004;7(3):157–63.

48. Rajasekaran S, Vanderpump M, Baldeweg S, et al. UK guidelines for the management of pituitary apoplexy. Clin Endocrinol (Oxf) 2011;74(1):9–20.

49. Almeida JP, Sanchez MM, Karekezi C, et al. Pituitary apoplexy: results of surgical and conservative management clinical series and review of the literature. World Neurosurg 2019;130:e988–99.

Obesity

Tyler Fuller, MD[1], Zakary Newberry, MD[1], Munima Nasir, MD,
Justin Tondt, MD*

KEYWORDS

- Obesity • BMI • Diet • Exercise • Bariatric surgery

KEY POINTS

- Obesity is a complex, multifactorial disease that is highly prevalent in the United States.
- Evaluation of obesity includes a thorough history and physical examination as well as basic laboratory tests for complications and secondary causes.
- Treatment of obesity involves a multidisciplinary approach for lifestyle interventions, and when appropriate, pharmacotherapy and surgical interventions.

INTRODUCTION

The Obesity Medicine Association defines obesity as "a chronic, progressive, relapsing, and treatable multifactorial, neuro-behavioral disease, wherein an increase in body fat promotes adipose tissue dysfunction and abnormal fat mass physical forces, resulting in adverse metabolic, biomechanical, and psychosocial health consequences."[1] Clinically, obesity is often defined by body mass index (BMI) of $\geq$30 in adults or $\geq$95th percentile for age in children. Obesity can be further subdivided into class I, class II, and class III, as shown in **Table 1**.[2] Of note, the Centers for Disease Control and Prevention extended BMI-For-Age growth charts are needed to differentiate class II and class III obesity in children. Several other diagnostic criteria for obesity exist, including waist circumference, body fat percentage, Edmonton obesity staging system, and American Association of Clinical Endocrinologists (AACE) obesity staging system.[3,4] While each of these have advantages, they are less commonly used than BMI.

Obesity results from a multifactorial and complex interplay between physiologic, behavioral, and environmental factors. On a hormonal level, ghrelin, produced in the stomach, stimulates hunger whereas glucagon-like peptide 1 and multiple other hormones produced in the small intestine, large intestine, and pancreas contribute to episodic satiety and leptin secreted from adipose tissue contributes to tonic satiety.[5]

Department of Family and Community Medicine, Penn State University College of Medicine, Milton S. Hershey Medical Center, 700 HMC Crescent Road, Hershey, PA 17033, USA
[1] Shared first authorship.
* Corresponding author.
E-mail address: jtondt1@pennstatehealth.psu.edu

Prim Care Clin Office Pract 51 (2024) 511–522
https://doi.org/10.1016/j.pop.2024.04.007
0095-4543/24/© 2024 Elsevier Inc. All rights reserved.

Table 1
Definitions of class I, class II, and class III obesity in adults and children

	Body Mass Index—Adults	Body Mass Index for Age—Pediatrics
Class I obesity	30–34	100%–119% of 95th percentile
Class II obesity	35–39	120%–139% of 95th percentile
Class III obesity	≥ 40	≥140% of 95th percentile

$$Body\ Mass\ Index = \frac{body\ weight\ in\ kilograms}{(height\ in\ meters)^2}$$

These hormonal factors are integrated in the hypothalamus along with input from the vagus nerve, frontal cortex, limbic system, and other factors to regulate appetite.[5] In obesity, this finely balanced system is dysfunctional, leading to increased appetite, decreased energy expenditure, and the accumulation of excess adipose tissue.[6]

Obesity is one of the most common chronic diseases in the United States. Over 41% of adults over the age of 20 were classified as obese from 2017 to 2020.[7] There are over 200 obesity-associated disorders affecting almost all body systems. Obesity is well known to have adverse impacts on the cardiovascular system, including an increased risk of hypertension, coronary artery disease, myocardial infarction, congestive heart failure, atrial fibrillation, and stroke.[8–13] Diabetes is also strongly associated with obesity, with greater than 80% of type 2 diabetes being attributed to obesity.[14] Nonalcoholic fatty liver disease is strongly associated with obesity as well and is now one of the most common indications for liver failure and transplantation in the United States.[15]

Furthermore, obesity is associated with social determinants of health. Rates of obesity are higher in Black and Hispanic adults compared to Caucasian and Asian adults, and these trends are mirrored in childhood obesity.[16] Across all races, adult women have higher rates of obesity than adult men of the same race or ethnicity. Relative to household income, women experience higher rates of obesity with more poverty and less education, whereas men have rates of obesity in middle incomes and moderate education.[17]

EVALUATION

The US Preventive Services Task Force (USPSTF) recommends screening all children 6 years and older, adolescents, and adults for obesity.[18,19] However, when diagnosing obesity, it is important to recognize that patients with obesity are frequently exposed to obesity stigma and bias, even in health care settings. In order to reduce this bias, providers can utilize strategies such as reflecting on personal biases, using nonjudgmental and people-first language, and creating supportive office environments including wide and sturdy chairs, large gowns and blood pressure cuffs, and private weighing locations.[20]

In the evaluation of obesity, a thorough history pertaining to the patient's body weight is essential. This should include the pattern of body weight gain over a patient's lifetime as well as factors that influence a patient's change in weight, including physical and mental health, medications, surgery, and life circumstances. Family history can be beneficial in identifying familial metabolic diseases and assessing a patient's risk of cardiovascular disease. An important aspect of a patient's history as it relates to obesity is their nutrition history. This includes the food and beverages the patient consumes on a daily basis, the behavior the patient exhibits around eating, and previous nutritional attempts to lose weight. Physical examination should include vital signs, height, weight, waist circumference, and neck circumference, as well as examining for signs of Cushing's disease, polycystic ovarian syndrome (PCOS), goiter, and acanthosis nigricans.[21]

Laboratory evaluation should include a comprehensive metabolic panel (CMP), hemoglobin A1c (HbA1c), lipid profile, and thyroid-stimulating hormone (TSH). These should be acquired to assess comorbidities often associated with obesity including type 2 diabetes mellitus, dyslipidemia, and nonalcoholic fatty liver disease, as well as to evaluate for secondary causes of obesity such as hypothyroidism. Further evaluation can be performed on an individualized basis with body composition analysis, insulin levels, sex hormone levels, cortisol levels, vitamin levels, electrocardiography, and polysomnography.[21]

THERAPEUTIC OPTIONS

Treatment of obesity involves a multidisciplinary approach, including nutrition, physical activity, behavioral therapy, pharmacotherapy, and surgical intervention. The USPSTF recommends that patients with a BMI of 30 or higher be referred for intensive, multicomponent behavioral intervention and the AACE/American College of Endocrinology recommends intensifying behavioral therapy strategies if a 2.5% weight reduction is not achieved in the first month, citing that weight loss in the first month is a strong predictor of long-term weight loss.[19,22] Adherence to lifestyle changes is critical for weight loss prevention or weight regain. Patients often find that supervised visits facilitate accountability, and having frequent office visits with a multidisciplinary team that may include obesity specialists, dietitians, educators, and trainers can enhance the success of behavioral therapy.[22,23] The USPSTF has found that 26 or more contact hours in a year is significantly associated with more significant weight loss.[18]

Dietary interventions typically center around calorie restriction, meal timing, macronutrient-based dietary modifications, and overall dietary patterns.[24] There is strong evidence supporting dietary approaches with formal caloric prescription as well as dietary approaches with elimination of certain foods.[25] All dietary approaches rely on achieving a total cumulative energy deficit, even if calorie restriction is not the explicit intervention.[24,25] However, calorie restriction alone does not account for hunger, and counseling on food choices to promote satiety may improve adherence. If providing a caloric prescription, then energy expenditure estimators, many of which are freely available on the Internet, can be used to target the deficit needed for a desired rate of weight loss. A deficit of 3500 kcal per week is commonly used to roughly estimate 1 lb of fat loss, but it is important to keep in mind that weight includes more factors than just fat and that weight loss is a dynamic process, so energy expenditure estimates need to be frequently updated.[26,27] The goal body weight loss is at least 5% for health benefits or more as mutually agreed upon with the patient. **Table 2** provides examples of commonly used dietary interventions for obesity.

Physical activity is another crucial lifestyle intervention used to promote weight loss but is most beneficial when combined with dietary changes. Physical activity includes both planned exercise activities (exercise activity thermogenesis or EAT) to improve health as well as daily activities such as ambulation and leisure activities (Non-EAT or NEAT).[28] EAT can be written as an exercise prescription (**Table 3**) for either aerobic or anaerobic activity and may involve exercise physiologists as part of the multidisciplinary team.[22] NEAT can also be modified to help promote weight loss and a healthy lifestyle by decreasing sedentary time.[28]

Table 2
Examples of dietary interventions for obesity

Diet	Definition	Effect
VLCD	Limits energy intake to<800 kcal/day.[24]	This diet promotes rapid weight loss; there is insufficient evidence supporting better long-term weight loss and maintenance compared to other energy-restrictive diets.[24,28] VLCDs are associated with other effects, including lowering blood sugar and blood pressure, and it is important to have clinician supervision to ensure appropriate blood glucose and blood pressure control.[25]
Low-fat	<30% of daily calories from fat.[24,28]	This diet along with concurrent energy restriction was shown to promote weight loss compared to placebo.[24,25,28]
LCD	Daily carbohydrate restriction<130g.[29]	LCDs showed weight loss compared to placebo, especially in short-term (<6 mo) studies. LCDs showed more significant weight loss in the first 6 months compared to LFDs, but after 1–2 y, the weight loss was similar to LFDs and other calorie-restricted diets.[24,25]
Ketogenic	This is a very LCD that aims to induce ketosis to promote weight loss.[24,28]	It is similarly effective for promoting weight loss as other LCDs.[24]
Mediterranean	Encourages the consumption of olive oils, certain nuts, and vegetables that discourage the consumption of red meats and ultra-processed carbohydrates.	This has proven cardiovascular benefits and when combined with energy restriction, weight loss.[25]
Vegetarian	Primarily centered around avoiding meats. Some variations of vegetarian diets allow the consumption of eggs and/or fish, whereas others avoid all animal products, including dairy.	It can be associated with weight loss when including healthful, natural, plant-based foods.[28] Still, these benefits can be nullified when the diet includes unhealthful, high-calorie, processed foods.[28,30]

(continued on next page)

Table 2
(continued)

Diet	Definition	Effect
Intermittent fasting	Alternation of days with normal feeding and days of fasting.[28]	These diets have shown similar weight loss as continuous energy restriction and can be an effective strategy for weight loss for certain patients.[24]
Time-restricted feeding	Normal feeding is only limited to a few hours a day, typically 8 hours, and the individual limits their food intake for the remaining hours.[24]	

Abbreviations: LCD, low-carbohydrate diets; LFD, low-fat diet; VLCD, very–low-calorie diet.

The recommended physical activity per week for all adults is 150 to 300 minutes of moderate-intensity physical activity or 75 to 150 minutes of vigorous-intensity physical activity as well as at least 2 sessions of muscle-strengthening activity.[32] Moderate-intensity physical activity between 150 and 250 minutes per week effectively prevents weight gain but provides only modest weight loss.[33] Greater than 250 minutes per week of physical activity is associated with clinically significant weight loss and improved weight maintenance.[33] This type of physical activity does not enhance weight loss but resistance training may simultaneously increase fat-free mass and loss of fat mass, and any type of physical activity even without weight loss improves health outcomes.[33] In patients with obesity, physical activity with weight loss can also provide additional benefits, such as improving sleep apnea, osteoarthritis, and insulin sensitivity, as well as cardiopulmonary and mental health.[22,28]

Although behavioral modifications include nutrition and physical activity, behavioral treatment strategies, such as self-monitoring, motivational interviewing, and cognitive restructuring, can be used to improve adherence.[34] Self-monitoring weight, food intake, and/or physical activity can help promote mindfulness and improve the clinician's ability to identify areas for further intervention.[23] Motivational interviewing creates a patient-centered and goal-directed approach to help use the patient's own motivation to fuel positive lifestyle modifications.[23,34] Cognitive restructuring attempts to replace disadvantageous thoughts (overgeneralization, all-or-nothing thinking, and emotional reasoning) with more advantageous thoughts, and mental health providers may facilitate this in patients with eating disorders or other comorbid mental health conditions.[22,23,34]

Pharmacotherapy combined with lifestyle interventions has been shown to increase weight loss compared to lifestyle interventions alone.[6,11] Pharmacotherapy should only be used as an adjunct to lifestyle modifications and in patients with a BMI $\geq$ 30 alone or $\geq$ 27 with an obesity comorbidity.[35] Still, it may also increase adherence to behavioral interventions and more rapidly increase physical functioning to make exercise more feasible for patients.[35] The choice of pharmacologic agent for weight loss should be individualized to the patient considering their medical history and the medication characteristics.[22,35] **Table 4** shows the Food and Drug Administration–approved medications for obesity, which include orlistat, liraglutide, semaglutide, tirzepatide, phentermine, phentermine-topiramate, and bupropion-naltrexone. All of these are approved for long-term use except for phentermine, which is only approved for short-term use but commonly used off-label for long-term use. Of note, orlistat, liraglutide, semaglutide, and phentermine-topiramate are approved for ages 12 years and older whereas phentermine is approved for ages 17 years and older and

Table 3
Example exercise prescription

Fitte or FITT-VP[31] Acronym	Definition	Example
Frequency	How often?	3–5 times weekly
Intensity	How hard?	Moderate–vigorous.
Time spent	Duration	30–60 min
Type	What activity?	Aerobic
Enjoyment level	How much do you enjoy it?	Sports, competition, utilizing music
Volume	Total volume (amount) of exercise	2.5–5 h total weekly
Progression	Advancement of exercise program	Start by slowly progressing activity level and duration until at goal

bupropion-naltrexone is approved for ages 18 years and older. None of these medications have been extensively studied in a geriatric population. The goal body weight loss with any medication is at least 5% by 12 weeks.

From the primary care perspective, it is paramount to recognize which patients are candidates for surgery. Traditionally, bariatric surgery has been considered for patients with a BMI greater than 40 kg/m^2 and for those with a BMI greater than 35 kg/m^2 plus adverse effects of obesity (ie, diabetes, hypertension, obstructive sleep apnea).[40] In 2022, the American Society for Metabolic and Bariatric Surgery released new recommendations for bariatric surgery as an option for patients (without coexisting medical problems) with a BMI greater than 35 kg/m^2 and for patients with a BMI greater than 30 kg/m^2 plus obesity-related comorbidities or who have failed nonoperative weight loss measures.[41,42] Of note, for Asian individuals, the BMI threshold is lower at 27.5 kg/m2.[41] Currently, the most common bariatric surgery procedures are Roux-en-Y gastric bypass and vertical sleeve gastrectomy as laparoscopic adjustable gastric banding has fallen out of favor. After potential candidates are identified, there is an extensive education and evaluation process typically performed by bariatric surgery programs themselves prior to determining surgical eligibility. It is important to note that bariatric surgery should not replace dietary changes, physical activity, behavioral therapy, and medication management, but rather be combined with these interventions.[40]

DISCUSSION

Obesity is a complex, multifactorial disease that is highly prevalent in the United States and is associated with many disorders, including cardiovascular disease, diabetes, and liver disease. The USPSTF recommends screening all patients older than 6 years old for obesity. Patients with obesity frequently experience stigma and bias necessitating a sensitive approach during screening and management.

Obesity is typically classified by BMI. Assessment includes an in-depth history that includes medical, surgical, nutritional, behavioral, social, and familial as well as an in-depth physical examination that includes vitals, BMI, waist circumference, neck circumference, and signs of Cushing's disease, PCOS, and hypothyroidism. Initial evaluation should also include CMP, HbA1c, lipid panel, and TSH.

Treatment of obesity involves a multidisciplinary approach. Nutrition, physical activity, behavioral therapy, pharmacotherapy, and surgical intervention are all important

Table 4
Pharmacotherapy for obesity

Medication	Mechanism	Precautions[b] and Side Effects	Considerations
Orlistat Weight loss in excess of placebo[a]: 3%	Gastrointestinal lipase inhibitor that stimulates weight loss by inducing fat malabsorption.[36]	Contraindication: chronic malabsorption syndrome, oxalate nephropathy, or cholestasis. Side effects: oily stool and fecal incontinence.[22,36]	Consider in patients with cardiovascular disease as its benefits include reducing cardiovascular risks (improves blood pressure and lipid levels).[22,35,37]
Liraglutide Weight loss in excess of placebo[a]: 5%	GLP-1 receptor agonist promotes satiety.[36]	Contraindication: personal or family history of medullary thyroid carcinoma, multiple endocrine neoplasia type 2. Side effects: nausea, vomiting, diarrhea, constipation, flatulence, GERD, fatigue, headache, and dizziness.[36]	Can improve glycemic control and reduce the risk of major adverse cardiovascular events in patients with type 2 diabetes.[35,36] In addition to improving the effects noted for liraglutide, semaglutide also reduces the risk of major adverse cardiovascular events in patients with obesity and established cardiovascular disease without diabetes.[35,36,38] Greater weight reduction than liraglutide.[36]
Semaglutide Weight loss in excess of placebo[a]: 13%			
Tirzepatide Weight loss in excess of placebo[a]: 18%	Dual GIP/GLP-1 receptor agonist, although the GIP may mimic antagonism.[36]		Greater weight reduction than semaglutide.[39]
Phentermine Weight loss in excess of placebo[a]: 5%	Noradrenergic sympathomimetic amine that augments weight loss by reducing appetite.[35,36]	Contraindication: uncontrolled hypertension, heart disease, and hyperthyroidism.[35,36] Side effects: tremors, increased heart rate and blood pressure, dry mouth, headaches, and insomnia. Interacts with monoamine oxidase inhibitors, anti-hypertensives, adrenergic neuron blockers, and hypoglycemic medications.[36]	Low-cost medication approved for short-term weight loss but is often used off label for long-term weight management.[36]

(continued on next page)

Table 4
(continued)

Medication	Mechanism	Precautions[b] and Side Effects	Considerations
Phentermine-topiramate Weight loss in excess of placebo[a]: 7%–8%	Noradrenergic sympathomimetic amine combined with neurostabilizer which increases appetite suppression of phentermine alone by an unclear mechanism.[35–37]	Side effects: In addition to the side effects of phentermine alone, side effects of topiramate include metabolic acidosis, drowsiness, nephrolithiasis, constipation, dysgeusia, and paresthesia.[36] Pregnancy monitoring for reproductive age females taking topiramate due to an increased risk of oral clefts.[36]	Combination medication that is approved for chronic weight management. Topiramate should be slowly tapered to decrease seizure risk when stopping.[37]
Bupropion-naltrexone Weight loss in excess of placebo[a]: 5%	Antidepressant (norepinephrine and dopamine reuptake inhibitor) and an opioid antagonist that augments weight loss by stimulating neurons that promote satiety.[35]	Contraindication: uncontrolled hypertension, seizure disorders, and opioid use.[22,36,37] Side effects: headache, insomnia, dry mouth, and GI distress (nausea, constipation, vomiting, diarrhea).[36]	Consider in patients with depression or who are seeking smoking cessation.

Abbreviations: GERD, gastroesophageal reflux disease; GI, gastrointestinal; GIP, glucose-dependent insulinotropic polypeptide; GLP-1, glucagon-like peptide 1.
[a] Placebo group ranges from 2% to 6% body weight loss depending on the specific study.
[b] Pregnancy and hypersensitivity are contraindications for all listed medications.

aspects of treating obesity. Adherence to all lifestyle changes is paramount for weight loss. Total cumulative energy deficit is the basis of most dietary interventions and is recommended for successful weight loss. Physical activity is most beneficial for weight loss when combined with the aforementioned nutritional changes. Frequent supervised visits, self-monitoring, and goal setting are all behavioral strategies used to facilitate weight loss. Referral to a multidisciplinary team can facilitate these lifestyle interventions. Weight loss medications can be helpful as adjuncts to lifestyle interventions. Surgical management of weight loss can be considered in patients with a BMI greater than 40 kg/m^2 or greater than 35 kg/m^2 with comorbidities.

Future directions will likely include a more individualized evaluation and treatment of obesity. BMI is the primary measurement used to classify obesity, but may not accurately measure body fat for every individual.[43] Waist circumference and body fat composition analysis have been emerging as additional measurements of obesity. Furthermore, treatments that preferentially target fat mass, specifically visceral fat mass, while minimizing loss of lean body mass are an important topic of future study. As technological advances continue to be made, digital and remote options are likely to become increasingly common.

CLINICS CARE POINTS

- The USPSTF recommends screening all patients 6 years or older for obesity and treating with multicomponent, intensive behavioral interventions.
- Obesity is typically classified BMI 30 or more in adults and 95th percentile or more in children.
- Nonjudgmental, person-first language is important to perpetuating obesity bias and stigma.
- Initial evaluation of obesity includes a thorough history and physical examination as well as laboratory testing for blood glucose, liver function, lipids, and thyroid function.
- Multiple dietary interventions are effective for weight loss by either directly or indirectly reducing calorie intake.
- Physical activity is often only modestly effective for weight loss but has additional health benefits that support its use.
- Motivational interviewing, cognitive behavioral therapy, and other behavioral strategies are important components to promote adherence.
- Several medications are indicated for patients with a BMI $\geq$ 30 or $\geq$27 with an obesity comorbidity.
- Bariatric surgery referral is indicated for patients with a BMI $\geq$ 40 or $\geq$ 35 with an obesity comorbidity.

DISCLOSURE

The authors have no conflicts of interest to disclose.

REFERENCES

1. Tondt J, Freshwater M, Christensen S, et al. Obesity algorithm ebook, presented by the obesity medicine association. www.obesityalgorithm.org. Published 2023. Available at: https://obesitymedicine.org/obesity-algorithm/.
2. Clinical guidelines on the identification, evaluation, and treatment of overweight and obesity in adults–the evidence report. National Institutes of health. Obes Res 1998;6(Suppl 2):51S–209S.

3. Padwal R, Leslie WD, Lix LM, et al. Relationship among body fat percentage, body mass index, and all-cause mortality: a cohort study. Ann Intern Med 2016;164(8):532–41.

4. Alberti KGMM, Zimmet P, Shaw J. Metabolic syndrome–a new world-wide definition. A Consensus Statement from the International Diabetes Federation. Diabet Med J Br Diabet Assoc 2006;23(5):469–80.

5. Benelam B. Satiation, satiety and their effects on eating behaviour. Nutr Bull 2009; 34(2):126–73.

6. Perry B, Wang Y. Appetite regulation and weight control: the role of gut hormones. Nutr Diabetes 2012;2(1):e26.

7. Stierman B, Joseph A, Margaret C, et al. NHSR 158. National Health and Nutrition Examination Survey 2017–March 2020 Pre-Pandemic Data Files. National Center for Health Statistics (U.S.) 2021. https://doi.org/10.15620/cdc:106273.

8. Wilson PWF, D'Agostino RB, Sullivan L, et al. Overweight and obesity as determinants of cardiovascular risk: the Framingham experience. Arch Intern Med 2002; 162(16):1867–72.

9. Bogers RP, Bemelmans WJE, Hoogenveen RT, et al. Association of overweight with increased risk of coronary heart disease partly independent of blood pressure and cholesterol levels: a meta-analysis of 21 cohort studies including more than 300 000 persons. Arch Intern Med 2007;167(16):1720–8.

10. Kenchaiah S, Evans JC, Levy D, et al. Obesity and the risk of heart failure. N Engl J Med 2002;347(5):305–13.

11. Yusuf S, Hawken S, Ounpuu S, et al. Obesity and the risk of myocardial infarction in 27,000 participants from 52 countries: a case-control study. Lancet Lond Engl 2005;366(9497):1640–9.

12. Wang TJ, Parise H, Levy D, et al. Obesity and the risk of new-onset atrial fibrillation. JAMA 2004;292(20):2471–7.

13. Towfighi A, Zheng L, Ovbiagele B. Weight of the obesity epidemic: rising stroke rates among middle-aged women in the United States. Stroke 2010;41(7): 1371–5.

14. Colditz GA, Willett WC, Rotnitzky A, et al. Weight gain as a risk factor for clinical diabetes mellitus in women. Ann Intern Med 1995;122(7):481–6.

15. Tarantino G, Saldalamacchia G, Conca P, et al. Non-alcoholic fatty liver disease: further expression of the metabolic syndrome. J Gastroenterol Hepatol 2007; 22(3):293–303.

16. Ogden CL, Fakhouri TH, Carroll MD, et al. Prevalence of obesity among adults, by household income and education - United States, 2011-2014. MMWR Morb Mortal Wkly Rep 2017;66(50):1369–73.

17. Hales CM, Carroll MD, Fryar CD, et al. Prevalence of obesity and severe obesity among adults: United States, 2017-2018. NCHS Data Brief 2020;(360):1–8.

18. US Preventive Services Task Force. Screening for obesity in children and adolescents: US preventive services task force recommendation statement. JAMA 2017;317(23):2417–26.

19. US Preventive Services Task Force. Behavioral weight loss interventions to prevent obesity-related morbidity and mortality in adults: US preventive services task force recommendation statement. JAMA 2018;320(11):1163–71.

20. Fruh SM, Nadglowski J, Hall HR, et al. Obesity stigma and bias. J Nurse Pract JNP 2016;12(7):425.

21. Panuganti KK, Nguyen M, Kshirsagar RK. Obesity. In: StatPearls. StatPearls Publishing; 2023. Available at: http://www.ncbi.nlm.nih.gov/books/NBK459357/. [Accessed 24 November 2023].

22. Garvey WT, Mechanick JI, Brett EM, et al. American Association of Clinical Endocrinologists and American College of Endocrinology Comprehensive Clinical Practice Guidelines for Medical Care of Patients with Obesity. Endocr Pract Off J Am Coll Endocrinol Am Assoc Clin Endocrinol 2016;22(Suppl 3):1–203.

23. Freshwater M, Christensen S, Oshman L, et al. Behavior, motivational interviewing, eating disorders, and obesity management technologies: An Obesity Medicine Association (OMA) Clinical Practice Statement (CPS) 2022. Obes Pillars 2022;2:100014.

24. Chao AM, Quigley KM, Wadden TA. Dietary interventions for obesity: clinical and mechanistic findings. J Clin Invest 2021;131(1):e140065, 140065.

25. Jensen MD, Ryan DH, Apovian CM, et al. 2013 AHA/ACC/TOS Guideline for the Management of Overweight and Obesity in Adults. Circulation 2014; 129(25_suppl_2):S102–38.

26. Thomas DM, Gonzalez MC, Pereira AZ, et al. Time to correctly predict the amount of weight loss with dieting. J Acad Nutr Diet 2014;114(6):857–61.

27. Hall K, Chow C. Why is the 3500 kcal per pound weight loss rule wrong? Int J Obes 2005;37(12). 2013.

28. Alexander L, Christensen SM, Richardson L, et al. Nutrition and physical activity: An Obesity Medicine Association (OMA) Clinical Practice Statement 2022. Obes Pillars 2022;1:100005.

29. Feinman RD, Pogozelski WK, Astrup A, et al. Dietary carbohydrate restriction as the first approach in diabetes management: Critical review and evidence base. Nutrition 2015;31(1):1–13.

30. Hall KD, Ayuketah A, Brychta R, et al. Ultra-processed diets cause excess calorie intake and weight gain: an inpatient randomized controlled trial of ad libitum food intake. Cell Metabol 2019;30(1):67–77.e3.

31. Bushman BA. Determining the I (Intensity) for a FITT-VP aerobic exercise prescription. ACSM's Health & Fit J 2014;18(3):4.

32. Piercy KL, Troiano RP, Ballard RM, et al. The physical activity guidelines for Americans. JAMA 2018;320(19):2020–8.

33. Donnelly JE, Blair SN, Jakicic JM, et al, American College of Sports Medicine Position Stand. Appropriate physical activity intervention strategies for weight loss and prevention of weight regain for adults. Med Sci Sports Exerc 2009;41(2): 459–71.

34. Burgess E, Hassmén P, Welvaert M, et al. Behavioural treatment strategies improve adherence to lifestyle intervention programmes in adults with obesity: a systematic review and meta-analysis. Clin Obes 2017;7(2):105–14.

35. Apovian CM, Aronne LJ, Bessesen DH, et al. Pharmacological management of obesity: an endocrine Society clinical practice guideline. J Clin Endocrinol Metab 2015;100(2):342–62.

36. Bays HE, Fitch A, Christensen S, et al. Anti-Obesity Medications and Investigational Agents: An Obesity Medicine Association (OMA) Clinical Practice Statement (CPS) 2022. Obes Pillars 2022;2:100018.

37. Erlandson M, Ivey LC, Seikel K. Update on office-based strategies for the management of obesity. Am Fam Physician 2016;94(5):361–8.

38. Lincoff AM, Brown-Frandsen K, Colhoun HM, et al. Semaglutide and Cardiovascular Outcomes in Obesity without Diabetes. N Engl J Med 2023;0(0). https://doi.org/10.1056/NEJMoa2307563. null.

39. Jastreboff AM, Aronne LJ, Ahmad NN, et al. Tirzepatide once weekly for the treatment of obesity. N Engl J Med 2022;387(3):205–16.

40. Shetye B, Hamilton FR, Bays HE. Bariatric surgery, gastrointestinal hormones, and the microbiome: An Obesity Medicine Association (OMA) Clinical Practice Statement (CPS) 2022. Obes Pillars 2022;2:100015.

41. Eisenberg D, Shikora SA, Aarts E, et al. 2022 American Society for Metabolic and Bariatric Surgery (ASMBS) and International Federation for the Surgery of Obesity and Metabolic Disorders (IFSO): Indications for Metabolic and Bariatric Surgery. Surg Obes Relat Dis 2022;18(12):1345–56.

42. Mechanick JI, Youdim A, Jones DB, et al. Clinical practice guidelines for the peri-operative nutritional, metabolic, and nonsurgical support of the bariatric surgery patient–2013 update: cosponsored by American Association of Clinical Endocri-nologists, the Obesity Society, and American Society for Metabolic & Bariatric Surgery. Endocr Pract Off J Am Coll Endocrinol Am Assoc Clin Endocrinol 2013;19(2):337–72.

43. Bays HE, Golden A, Tondt J. Thirty Obesity Myths, Misunderstandings, and/or Oversimplifications: An Obesity Medicine Association (OMA) Clinical Practice Statement (CPS) 2022. Obes Pillars 2022;3:100034.

Sports Endocrinology

Henry Lau, DO[a], Tyler M. Janitz, DO[b], Alec Sikarin, MD[a],
Ramla N. Kasozi, MB, ChB, MPH[b],*, George G.A. Pujalte, MD[b],*

KEYWORDS

- Sports • Endocrine • Female athlete • Bone health • Osteoporosis • Osteopenia
- Exercise • Diabetes

KEY POINTS

- Exercise has important health benefits for patients with diabetes but can also increase the risk of hypoglycemia.
- Strategies to adapt to exercise such as monitoring blood sugar, adjusting medications, and increasing carbohydrate intake are essential in patients with diabetes.
- Relative energy deficiency in sports is the new terminology for the Female Athlete Triad, which involves menstrual irregularity, low bone mineral density (BMD), and low energy availability in female athletes.
- Pharmacotherapy is typically not recommended for premenopausal athletes who have low BMD without a history of fractures or identified secondary causes of low BMD.
- Discussion of performance enhancing drugs should be part of wellness exams or sports physicals with athletes.

INTRODUCTION TO SPORTS ENDOCRINOLOGY

Sports endocrinology holds a unique importance in understanding and optimizing an active and healthy lifestyle. This special area of endocrinology focuses on the intricate hormonal responses that occur during exercise, training, and recovery, thus influencing various physiologic processes critical to physical activity and athletic training. This area of medicine is very broad with entire textbooks dedicated to it. This article will focus on the effects of exercise on blood sugar and diabetes, bone health, and topics unique to female athletes.

Exercise has a considerable impact on blood sugar levels. Physical activity enhances insulin sensitivity, allowing cells to better use glucose. Regular exercise helps regulate blood sugar, reducing the risk of diabetes, and managing the condition in those already diagnosed. Exercise has a significant impact on blood sugar. Therefore,

[a] Department of Family Medicine, Tidelands Health, 4320 Holmestown Road, Myrtle Beach, SC 29588, USA; [b] Department of Family Medicine, Mayo Clinic, 4500 San Pablo Road, Jacksonville, FL 32224, USA
* Corresponding authors.
E-mail addresses: Kasozi.Ramla@mayo.edu (R.N.K.); pujalte.george@mayo.edu (G.G.A.P.)

Prim Care Clin Office Pract 51 (2024) 523–533
https://doi.org/10.1016/j.pop.2024.04.008
0095-4543/24/© 2024 Elsevier Inc. All rights reserved.

special considerations for monitoring and adjusting medications may be necessary during episodes of increased physical stress.

Exercise plays a crucial role in the management and prevention of osteoporosis. Weight-bearing and resistance exercises, such as walking, jogging, and strength training, stimulate bone formation and enhance bone density. These activities also improve balance and reduce the risk of falls. Osteoporosis management involves a multifaceted approach that includes weight training, healthy diet, supplements, and prescription medications.

Regular exercise can positively influence the menstrual cycle by reducing menstrual discomfort, improving mood, and promoting overall well-being. However, excessive exercise without adequate nutrition may lead to irregularities or amenorrhea. Differential diagnosis, workup, and treatment of menstrual irregularities will also be addressed in this article.

The Female Athlete Triad (AKA: relative energy deficiency in sports [RED-S]) is a complex health condition with disordered eating, menstrual dysfunction, and low bone mineral density (BMD). Female athletes, particularly in high-impact or aesthetic sports, may experience this syndrome. The role of a multidisciplinary team in the management and treatment of this complex syndrome is of paramount importance. Anabolic steroids and other performance enhancers are popular and have significant side effects and complications.

EXERCISE AND DIABETES

Exercise influences blood sugar management in patients with diabetes, with major implications for both short-term glucose control and long-term metabolic health.[1] Heightened reliance on carbohydrates during exercise, especially at higher intensities, necessitates efficient glucose usage and management. For patients with diabetes, this means that physical activity can effectively lower and stabilize blood glucose levels, thereby aiding in the overall management of diabetes.

Regular exercise improves glycemic control in patients with diabetes through several different mechanisms, including increased GLUT4 transporter activity, increased glycogen breakdown, increased insulin sensitivity, and glycogen supercompensation.

With new or extreme exercise regimens, caution must be taken in diabetics due to an increased risk for cardiovascular disease, exercise-induced hypoglycemia, and musculoskeletal injury. It is particularly important to educate diabetic patients receiving insulin or secretagogue therapy regarding monitoring glucose levels and adjusting carbohydrate intake or medications with exercise.

One of the central mechanisms of glucose metabolism during exercise is the activity of the GLUT4 transporter.[2] During physical activity, GLUT4 transporters increase in number on the muscle cell surface, facilitating glucose uptake from the bloodstream into muscle cells. This activity fuels muscles while simultaneously lowering blood glucose levels.

Exercise increases muscle glycogen breakdown, particularly with high intensity activities.[2] This glycogenolysis, in turn, results in increased blood glucose uptake to replenishing glycogen stores, thereby lowering glucose levels in the bloodstream. After exercise, muscles become more insulin sensitive, further improving blood glucose control.

Glycogen supercompensation is another important response to exercise.[2] Glycogen supercompensation occurs following exercise, when muscles are able to store more glycogen than they had prior to the exercise. This increased storage capacity is crucial, not only for storing energy for future exercise, but for stabilizing blood sugar levels in patients with diabetes. **Fig. 1** describes how regular physical activity, regardless of type, can lead to a more stable glucose metabolism and lower A1C values.[3]

Sports-related Diabetes Treatment Considerations

- For patients with high cardiovascular risk, greater than 30 year-old (y.o.), or a previously sedentary lifestyle consider exercise stress testing and medical optimization prior to initiation of an exercise regimen.[3]
- Patients can use aerobic exercise, resistance training, or a combination of both in their exercise regimen with similar benefits and low risk.[3]
- Encourage 150 to 300 minutes per week of moderate-intensity or 75 to 150 minutes per week of vigorous-intensity exercise (or equivalent combination) for substantial health benefits.[4]
- In patients with diabetes requiring insulin therapy, increased carbohydrate intake is the mainstay for reducing the incidence of induced hypoglycemia.[5]
  - If the exercise duration is greater than 60 minutes, a 20% to 50% decrease in insulin dosing adjustment is reasonable.[5,6]
  - A simple regimen for carbohydrate replacement is 30 g of carbohydrates per hour of exercise.[6]
  - Due to increased risk of exercise-induced hypoglycemia, sulfonylureas and glinides should be avoided in patients on a regular exercise regimen.
- Measure blood glucose 2 to 3× prior to exercise to establish a baseline and closely monitor changes.[3]
  - If below 70:
    - Eat 15 g of fast-acting carbohydrates and recheck blood glucose in 15 minutes; only initiate exercise if blood glucose is higher than 90.
  - If between 70 and 90:
    - Patients with type 1 diabetes should consume 15 g of fast-acting carbohydrates and recheck blood glucose in 15 minutes, resuming exercise when glucose is higher than 90.
    - Patients with type 2 diabetes should consume 15 to 30 g of fast-acting carbohydrates and either immediately resume exercising if accustomed to starting at that blood glucose level or wait and recheck in 15 minutes if unaccustomed.
- If between 90 and 270, exercise is typically safe.
- Higher than 270:

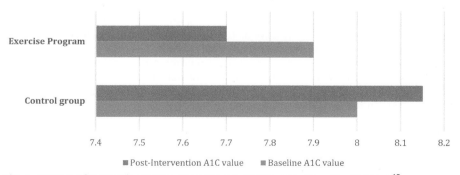

Fig. 1. Impact of 9 month exercise program on A1C in patients with diabetes.[13]

- Patients with type 2 diabetes should avoid exercise and medically address their hyperglycemia, either using short-acting insulin and measuring blood glucose 15 minutes later or seek medical attention, especially if symptomatic.
- Patients with type 1 diabetes should measure urine ketones and monitor for symptoms of diabetic ketoacidosis; they should seek emergency medical attention if one or more of the following are present with ketonuria.
  - Frequent urination and extreme thirst
  - Fatigue, weakness, or shortness of breath
  - Fruity-scented breath
  - Abdominal pain, nausea, or vomiting
  - Confusion

Summary

Overall, the physiologic changes induced by exercise offer substantial benefits for blood glucose regulation, particularly in diabetes. Through insulin-independent mediation reduction in blood glucose via the action of the GLUT4 transporter, increased glycogen use, glycogen supercompensation, and increased insulin sensitivity, exercise can effectively reduce hemoglobin A_{1c} and help reduce diabetic complications. Caution should be utilized when recommending exercise regimens to patients with diabetes, particularly those on insulin or insulin secretagogue therapy, with significant cardiac risk factors, long-standing diabetes, or a previously sedentary lifestyle.

BONE HEALTH FOR THE FEMALE ATHLETE

Introduction

While Sports Medicine involves the treatment of musculoskeletal injuries and performance optimization, it should also emphasize prevention and therapy for various orthopedic conditions. Low bone mineral density (BMD) is an important condition related to sports medicine and is more common in female athletes. Osteoporosis can increase the risk for injuries and significantly impact one's ability to stay active. While we traditionally think of athletes as young Olympic-caliber competitors, many Americans participate in athletic activities well into their seventh to eighth decade of life.

Osteoporosis is characterized by decreased BMD, structural deterioration of bone tissue, and heightened risk of fracture. Osteoporosis can be clinically diagnosed if an athlete has suffered a fragility fracture (even without measuring BMD) or if there is a T-score of −2.5 standard deviations (SDs), or lower at any site using dual energy x-ray absorptiometry (DEXA).

In the United States, a clinical diagnosis may also be based on the Fracture Risk Assessment Tool (FRAX), which estimates the risk of a major osteoporotic fracture over 10 years, but only for women over 40 years of age. Both a 10 year risk of major osteoporotic fracture of 20% or greater or 10 year risk of hip fracture 3% or greater are consider high FRAX scores.[7,8]

Osteoporosis is typically asymptomatic but can present with pain from fragility fractures that occur with low kinetic energy injuries or activities that typically would not cause a fracture. Fragility fractures typically occur in the spine, hip, and pelvis but can also occur in the wrist, rib, or humerus.[9]

Imaging

Imaging for the diagnosis and monitoring of osteoporosis is typically performed via DEXA.[9] A T-score of 1 to 2.5 SDs below the young adult average is classified as low bone mass, or osteopenia, and a T-score of 2.5 SDs or greater below the average is classified as osteoporosis.[7,8] The Z-score compares a patient's BMD to that of their age group. A Z-score of −2 or lower indicates a BMD that is significantly lower than expected for that age.[9] Pediatric athletes can be diagnosed with osteoporosis if they have either a vertebral compression fracture OR a Z-score less than −2 AND a history of significant fractures that occur with low energy sports injuries. Examples of qualifying significant fractures include 2 fractures of the long bones before 10 years of age or 3 such fractures before 19 years of age.

Approach for Premenopausal Athletes

Routine osteoporosis screening through BMD is generally not advised for premenopausal female athletes with the exception of those with known secondary causes for osteoporosis or a history of fragility fractures.[10] It is essential to evaluate and ensure calcium and vitamin D intake and levels and to assess exercise habits in all premenopausal women experiencing low bone mass. After reviewing medical history, physical examination, and initial laboratory test results, further testing and/or specialty referral may be necessary.

Generally, pharmacotherapy is not recommended for premenopausal athletes who only have low BMD without a history of fractures or identified secondary causes of low BMD. In those women, it is reasonable to ensure adequate calcium and vitamin D intake and schedule another BMD test in 1 to 2 years.[11,12] Women with a low BMD who show signs of continuing bone loss upon subsequent BMD assessments should be referred to a sports specialist with knowledge of metabolic bone conditions for further evaluation and treatment.[13]

Individuals with osteoporosis who experience fractures of the spine or hip and those with multiple fragility fractures should start pharmacologic treatment with BMD reassessment in 1 to 2 years.

There is a paucity of evidence to guide the pharmacologic treatment of premenopausal osteoporosis and referral to an endocrinologist, preferably with expertise in treating athletes, is recommended. For most premenopausal women with osteoporosis who qualify for pharmacologic treatment, starting bisphosphonates is recommended, with teriparatide as an alternative option.[14] Bisphosphonates and teriparatide can improve BMD in several types of premenopausal osteoporosis, but studies are small and do not provide evidence regarding fracture risk reduction. When considering the use of bisphosphonates or teriparatide for treating premenopausal osteoporosis, it is important to weigh the possible short-term and long-term risks, including those related to potential pregnancy.[15]

Approach for Postmenopausal Female Athletes

Postmenopausal female pharmacotherapy is recommended when osteoporosis is diagnosed due to a T-score of −2.5 or less, or a fragility fracture. If a treatable secondary cause is identified, it should be addressed accordingly. Additionally, postmenopausal women with a T-score between −1.0 and −2.5 and a high fracture risk might be considered for pharmacologic treatment, especially if their 10 year probability of a hip fracture or a major osteoporotic fracture is 3% or 20%, respectively. If the results show stable or improved BMD, the treatment should continue, and further BMD measurements can be taken every 2 to 5 years (depending on the clinical scenario).

Oral bisphosphonates are recommended as first-line treatment of postmenopausal female athletes with osteoporosis. Alendronate is often preferred because of its proven effectiveness in decreasing the risk of both vertebral and hip fractures, as well as evidence suggesting continued benefits in reducing fractures even after completing a 5 year treatment period.[16] Risedronate is as a suitable alternative to alendronate.[16]

Denosumab is a viable substitute for those who are not suitable for or cannot tolerate bisphosphonate therapy. This is often preferred over anabolic agents (teriparatide, abaloparatide, or romosozumab) for initial treatment.[16,17] For competitors unable to use oral bisphosphonates, intravenous bisphosphonates can be considered.[18]

There is some debate about the best initial treatment for active, postmenopausal women with a particularly high fracture risk, such as those with a T-score of −2.5 or lower and fragility fractures, a T-score of −3.0 or lower without fragility fractures, or a history of severe or numerous fractures. Some experts recommend starting with an anabolic agent due to its potent bone-building effects, while others favor bisphosphonates for initial treatment because anabolic agents are generally more costly, require subcutaneous injections, and have less long-term safety data available.

For sportswomen with a very high risk of fracture who did not start treatment with an anabolic agent, a switch to an anabolic therapy is recommended when initial treatment is ineffective.[19] After anabolic therapy is discontinued, patients should be treated with an antiresorptive agent (typically a bisphosphonate) to preserve the gains in BMD from anabolic therapy. For individuals who are unable to tolerate oral or intravenous bisphosphonates, denosumab, or raloxifene may be prescribed instead.[20]

THE FEMALE ATHLETE TRIAD (RED-S)
Introduction

A healthy high-performing female athlete has the necessary caloric intake to support energy demand and physiologic function while providing a sufficient balance between availability of energy in the form of calories, body function metabolism, and healthy menstrual cycle. In 2014, the International Olympic Committee changed the diagnostic definition from the female athlete triad to RED-S to adapt a more holistic view toward the pathologic diagnosis involving menstrual irregularity, low BMD, and low-energy availability.[21] Ultimately, low caloric energy intake or excessive caloric energy expenditure can cause maladaptive pathophysiologic and hormonal pathways that cause amenorrhea, improper bone development, and a variety of other signs and symptoms that lead to overall poor health outcomes.[11]

RED-S is usually seen in physically active girls and young women. It can occur in athletes of any sport and competition level, but is more common with gymnastics, figure skating, swimming, track and field, and rowing.[22,23] It is important for primary care physicians (PCPs) to identify athletes are risk for this triad so timely evaluation and interventions can be implemented.

Evaluation, Diagnosis, and Guidelines for RED-S

The overall incidence of RED-S is very ill defined for a variety of reasons including the variability of patient presentation and patient reluctance to provide a full, accurate history. It is important to recognize in evaluation that the athletes at highest risk for RED-S are those who participate in sports that emphasize a lean body structure and endurance, such as cheerleading, swimming, gymnastics, dance, and long-distance running.[24] The most common presenting symptoms include increased musculoskeletal injuries such as sprains and strains, infertility with menstrual irregularities, poor athletic performance due to decreased energy, and stress fractures secondary to low BMD. Due to these pathologies most commonly presenting in adolescence and early adulthood, the long-lasting effects of RED-S can include permanent infertility, lifelong disordered eating, osteoporosis, and psychiatric disease.[13] Recognition of those populations at highest risk of RED-S is essential to avoid these long-term life-altering presentations.

Screening and diagnosis of RED-S is very challenging as the symptoms can present slowly and subtly. However, a clinical assessment tool to assist medical professionals in identification and management does exist.[25] It is recommended that screening be completed as part of annual sports physicals and especially when an athlete presents with eating disorders, unusual weight loss, underweight body mass index, lack of normal growth or development, menstrual irregularity, or decreased sports performance of unclear cause.[26] If an athlete presents with these symptoms or there is high clinical suspicion based on patient presentation, it is recommended to undergo screening with laboratory and imaging workup.

The diagnosis of RED-S is largely clinical at first presentation with identification of the previously discussed phenotype and characteristics. However, based on clinical judgment of severity, further workup can be pursued by the clinician. Laboratory abnormalities that may be seen are consistent with decreased energy availability and hypogonadotropic hypogonadism including hypoglycemia, low leptin, low luteinizing hormone, low estrogen, low growth hormone, elevated cortisol, and decreased Z-score consistent with low BMD on DEXA.[27] If these laboratory abnormalities and symptoms of energy deficiency are present, it is recommended for the patient to continue training with a multidisciplinary treatment plan in place and follow-up every 1 to 3 months to assess compliance. Furthermore, if more serious features of disease such as anorexia nervosa, presence of extreme weight loss techniques leading to hemodynamic instability, or severe electrocardiography abnormalities such as bradycardia are present, that athlete should immediately cease all training with a written contract and begin a treatment program.[26]

Menstrual Disorders in RED-S

Menstrual disorders are a hallmark of RED-S. The most common menstrual disorders associated with sports are primary amenorrhea, secondary amenorrhea, and oligomenorrhea. The differential diagnosis is broad for these conditions, so ruling out other etiologies is essential.[28] Primary amenorrhea is defined as absence of the first menstrual period during normal development and evaluation for this disorder should occur if the patient has not menarche by 3 years after thelarche or by 15 y.o. or absent pubertal development by age of 13 years.[29] Secondary amenorrhea includes regular menses interrupted by the cessation of menses for 3 months or irregular menses interrupted for 6 months. Infrequent menses with intervals greater than 45 days in adolescent competitors and 35 days in adult athletes is oligomenorrhea.[30]

Evaluation of Amenorrhea

Evaluation of menstrual disorders in athletes is best done in consultation with a gynecologist. The most common causes of amenorrhea are structural, endocrine (eg, hypothalamic or pituitary disorders, primary ovarian insufficiency), sequelae of chronic diseases, or induced.[30] Initial laboratory testing includes ruling out pregnancy. In addition to a thorough history and physical examination, diagnostic tests are typically needed to determine the cause of amenorrhea. Serum total and free testosterone can be utilized to evaluate for hyperandrogenism. To assess endocrine etiologies, tests should include thyroid-stimulating hormone, prolactin, follicle-stimulating hormone, and luteinizing hormone. Elevated levels of anti-Mullerian hormone may indicate polycystic ovary syndrome or functional hypothalamic amenorrhea, while low levels indicate primary ovarian insufficiency rather than menopause. Transvaginal ultrasound can identify structural causes of amenorrhea (eg, polycystic, ovarian tumors) and MRI can be used to identify brain tumors.

Role of Primary Care and the Multidisciplinary Team

PCPs are uniquely positioned to educate patients, athletes, and coaches about RED-S during sports physicals and annual examinations. PCPs should be mindful of the common and subtle examination findings as they are most often the first medical professional patients present to for amenorrhea, fatigue, and musculoskeletal injuries. They should also be familiar with the clinical criteria and workup needed to diagnose the disease. It is imperative that PCPs educate colleagues about RED-S so it can be diagnosed more frequently and appropriately. Furthermore, PCPs can assist in changing the cultural barriers in sports and society that may lead to RED-S being underdiagnosed in the female athlete population.

Clinics Care Points

- There is little evidence to guide premenopausal osteoporosis and treatment should include referral to an endocrinologist or bone density specialist, preferably with expertise in treating athletes.
- Initial treatment of RED-S is typically non-pharmacologic and requires a multidisciplinary approach.
- Treatment of RED-S should focus on increasing energy intake through dietary changes and/or decreasing energy expenditure through training regimen modification.
- The overall goal of RED-S treatment is weight gain, increase in energy intake with decrease in expenditure, resumption of normal menses, and recovery of BMD.

PERFORMANCE ENHANCING DRUGS
Introduction

Performance enhancing drugs (PEDs) are agents used as an attempt to gain a competitive advantage. It has spread from professional sports to fitness and recreational sports. The majority of users are now recreational athletes.[31] Advantages may be in the form of increasing muscle mass and appearance in body building, strength in power lifting/explosive sports, and increased long distance performance in endurance sports such as triathlon. The World Anti-Doping Agency is the main organization that oversees policies and determines the list of substances and methods that are banned from competition.

PEDs include

1. Anabolic steroids, hormones that increase lean muscle mass, strength and decrease fat mass, are the most common used agents.[31]
2. Androgen precursors such as dehydroepiandrosterone (DHEA).
3. Human growth hormone (HCG).
4. Eythropoietin (EPO).

Discussion

Almost all androgens have been used as PEDs and include testosterone, trenbolone, 17-alpha androgen (oral), and boldnone (veterinary drug).[32] Most supplements can be purchased online or prescribed medically and legally such as testosterone for male hypogonadism. Some of the more potent steroids are procured through covert exchanges that are not regulated by the government or are purchased as veterinary grade medications.[33] Athletes will take these drugs as escalating doses over about 12 weeks (pyramiding) or by combining with 2 more steroids (stacking). Some stacks will include opposing drugs to counteract side effects, such as HCG with an anabolic to oppose testicular size reduction.[33]

DHEA is a precursor to testosterone and advertised in various fitness and body-building magazines. It is not androgenic but converted to testosterone and is touted to raise serum concentrations.[34]

HCG has effects on body composition as it increases muscle mass, strength, and greatly decreases fat. HCG binds to luteinizing hormone receptors and stimulates testes to secrete testosterone.[35]

EPO, which stimulates red blood cell production and thus increasing the oxygen carrying capacity, gained notoriety with the Tour de France. Prior to the popularity of EPO, athletes would train in hypoxic conditions such as at altitude and then transfusion their own blood prior to competition.[36]

Complications

While improving performance, there are many complications associated with these substances. Cardiac hypertrophy has been well documented in the literature with cases of sudden cardiac death due to myositis or hypertrophy.[37] Adverse effects on lipids such as major increase in low-density lipoprotein (LDL) and decrease in high-density lipoprotein (HDL) are well known.[38] Steroids have also been found to profoundly clotting factors leading to increased risk of thrombosis.[39] Severe erythropoiesis, leading to further risk of thrombus is also known.[40] Hypogonadism following discontinuation occurs in about 21% of men taking steroids.[41] Perhaps the most well-known complication is the neuropsychiatric side effects of severe aggression, depression, and even suicidal ideations.[41]

Summary

PEDs have made their way from professional into recreational sports. While there are many products on the market, the more well-known products are anabolic steroids, DHEA, HCG, and EPO. While they do enhance performance, there are many detrimental side effects and complications to their use.

CLINICS CARE POINTS

- Sports medicine physicians should have knowledge of the substances that are banned by various sporting organizations.
- Discussion of PEDs should be part of wellness examinations or sports physicals with athletes.
- Athletes who wish to stop using these substances should be encouraged but will need education that they will become temporarily hypogonadal.
- If athletes continue to use PEDs—cardiovascular, endocrine, hematopoietic, and psychiatric complications need to be considered and monitored.

DISCLOSURE

The authors have nothing to disclose.

REFERENCES

1. Jensen TE, Richter EA. Regulation of glucose and glycogen metabolism during and after exercise. J Physiol 2012;590:1069–76.
2. Colberg SR, Sigal RJ, Yardley JE, et al. Physical Activity/Exercise and Diabetes: A Position Statement of the American Diabetes Association. Diabetes Care 2016;39:2065–79.

3. Turner G, Quigg S, Davoren P, et al. Resources to Guide Exercise Specialists Managing Adults with Diabetes. Sports Med Open 2019;5:20.
4. Kanaley JA, Colberg SR, Corcoran MH, et al. Exercise/Physical Activity in Individuals with Type 2 Diabetes: A Consensus Statement from the American College of Sports Medicine. Med Sci Sports Exerc 2022;54:353–68.
5. Grimm JJ, Ybarra J, Berne C, et al. A new table for prevention of hypoglycaemia during physical activity in type 1 diabetic patients. Diabetes Metab 2004;30:465–70.
6. Cockcroft EJ, Narendran P, Andrews RC. Exercise-induced hypoglycaemia in type 1 diabetes. Exp Physiol 2020;105:590–9.
7. Cosman F, de Beur SJ, LeBoff MS, et al. Erratum to: Clinician's guide to prevention and treatment of osteoporosis. Osteoporos Int 2015;26:2045–7.
8. Cosman F, de Beur SJ, LeBoff MS, et al. Clinician's Guide to Prevention and Treatment of Osteoporosis. Osteoporos Int 2014;25:2359–81.
9. International Society for Clinical Densitometry. Official Positions. 2023. Available at: https://iscd.org/learn/official-positions/. [Accessed 22 January 2024].
10. Haseltine KN, Chukir T, Smith PJ, et al. Bone Mineral Density: Clinical Relevance and Quantitative Assessment. J Nucl Med 2021;62:446–54.
11. Cohen A, Shane E. Evaluation and management of the premenopausal woman with low BMD. Curr Osteoporos Rep 2013;11:276–85.
12. Haas AV, LeBoff MS. Osteoanabolic Agents for Osteoporosis. J Endocr Soc 2018;2:922–32.
13. Chamberlain R. The Female Athlete Triad: Recommendations for Management. Am Fam Physician 2018;97:499–502. Schmidt GA, Horner KE, McDanel DL, Ross MB, Moores.
14. Langdahl BL. Osteoporosis in premenopausal women. Curr Opin Rheumatol 2017;29(4):410–5.
15. Curtis EM, Reginster JY, Al-Daghri N, et al. Management of patients at very high risk of osteoporotic fractures through sequential treatments. Aging Clin Exp Res 2022;34:695–714.
16. Centre for Metabolic Bone Diseases. FRAX fracture risk assessment tool. University of Sheffield. Available at: https://frax.shef.ac.uk/FRAX/tool.aspx?country=9. Accessed January 22, 2024.
17. Walker MD, Shane E. Postmenopausal Osteoporosis. N Engl J Med 2023;389:1979–91.
18. Lewiecki EM, Bilezikian JP, Carey JJ, et al. Proceedings of the 2017 Santa Fe Bone Symposium: Insights and Emerging Concepts in the Management of Osteoporosis. J Clin Densitom 2018;21:3–21.
19. Miller PD. Clinical Management of Vertebral Compression Fractures. J Clin Densitom 2016;19:97–101.
20. International Society for Clinical Densitometry. Adult Official Positions. 2019. Available at: https://iscd.org/learn/official-positions/adult-positions/. [Accessed 22 January 2024].
21. Clark E, Tobias J. Metabolic and endocrine bone disorders. In: Blom A, Warwick D, Whitehouse M, editors. Apley & solomon's system of orthopaedics and trauma. 10th ed. Boca Raton: CRC Press; 2017. p. 121–55.
22. Matzkin E, Curry EJ, Whitlock K. Female Athlete Triad: Past, Present, and Future. J Am Acad Orthop Surg 2015;23:424–32.
23. De Souza MJ, Williams NI. Beyond hypoestrogenism in amenorrheic athletes: energy deficiency as a contributing factor for bone loss. Curr Sports Med Rep 2005;4:38–44.

24. De Souza MJ, Nattiv A, Joy E, et al. 2014 Female Athlete Triad Coalition consensus statement on treatment and return to play of the female athlete triad: 1st International Conference held in San Francisco, CA, May 2012, and 2nd International Conference held in Indianapolis, IN, May 2013. Clin J Sport Med 2014; 24:96–119.

25. Mountjoy M, Sundgot-Borgen J, Burke L, et al. The IOC consensus statement: beyond the Female Athlete Triad–Relative Energy Deficiency in Sport (RED-S). Br J Sports Med 2014;48:491–7.

26. Klein DA, Paradise SL, Reeder RM. Amenorrhea: A Systematic Approach to Diagnosis and Management. Am Fam Physician 2019;100:39–48.

27. Klein DA, Emerick JE, Sylvester JE, et al. Disorders of Puberty: An Approach to Diagnosis and Management. Am Fam Physician 2017;96:590–9.

28. Mauk KF, Clark BL. diagnosis, secreening, prevention, and treatement of osteoporosis. Mayo Clin Proc 2006;81:662–72.

29. Barrack M. Recommendations for Optimizing Bone Strength and Reducing Fracture Risk in Female Athletes. In: Beals KA, editor. Nutrition and the female athlete. 1st ed. Boca Raton: CRC Press; 2013. p. 229–46.

30. Cohn MR, Gianakos AL, Grueter K, et al. Update on the Comprehensive Approach to Fragility Fractures. J Orthop Trauma 2018;32:480–90.

31. Parkinson AB, Evans NA. Anabolic androgenic steroids: a survey of 500 users. Med Sci Sports Exerc 2006;38:644.

32. Pope HG Jr, Wood RI, Rogol A, et al. Adverse health consequences of performance-enhancing drugs: an Endocrine Society scientific statement. Endocr Rev 2014;35:341.

33. Rahnema CD, Lipshultz LI, Crosnoe LE, et al. Anabolic steroid-induced hypogonadism: diagnosis and treatment. Fertil Steril 2014;101:1271.

34. Morales AJ, Haubrich RH, Hwang JY, et al. The effect of six months treatment with a 100 mg daily dose of dehydroepiandrosterone (DHEA) on circulating sex steroids, body composition and muscle strength in age-advanced men and women. Clin Endocrinol 1998;49:421.

35. Handelsman DJ. Clinical review: The rationale for banning human chorionic gonadotropin and estrogen blockers in sport. J Clin Endocrinol Metab 2006;91: 1646.

36. Elliott S. Erythropoiesis-stimulating agents and other methods to enhance oxygen transport. Br J Pharmacol 2008;154:529.

37. Kennedy MC, Lawrence C. Anabolic steroid abuse and cardiac death. Med J Aust 1993;158:346.

38. Thompson PD, Cullinane EM, Sady SP, et al. Contrasting effects of testosterone and stanozolol on serum lipoprotein levels. JAMA 1989;261:1165.

39. Ferenchick GS, Hirokawa S, Mammen EF, et al. Anabolic-androgenic steroid abuse in weight lifters: evidence for activation of the hemostatic system. Am J Hematol 1995;49:282.

40. Stergiopoulos K, Brennan JJ, Mathews R, et al. Anabolic steroids, acute myocardial infarction and polycythemia: a case report and review of the literature. Vasc Health Risk Manag 2008;4:1475.

41. Knuth UA, Maniera H, Nieschlag E. Anabolic steroids and semen parameters in bodybuilders. Fertil Steril 1989;52:1041.

Endocrinology During Pregnancy

Sarah Inés Ramírez, MD, FAAFP[a],*, Elizabeth Ashley Suniega, MD[b],
Megan Ilene Laughrey, MD[b]

KEYWORDS

- Endocrine • Pregnancy • Postpartum • Diabetes • Thyroid • Placenta
- Social determinants

KEY POINTS

- Placental hormones regulate the reproductive axis, maternal metabolism, fetal growth, vasculogenesis, angiogenesis, and stress responses.
- Pregnancy is characterized by an increased risk of insulin resistance due to placental-produced hormones (ie, human placenta lactogen, progesterone, prolactin, placental growth hormone, cortisol) that increase throughout pregnancy and are greatest in the third trimester.
- In the first trimester, high concentrations of hCG results in weak stimulation of thyroid-stimulating hormone thereby stimulating the secretion of thyroid hormones.
- Social determinants of health are drivers of health outcomes representing almost 80% of the factors directly impacting the health of an individual.

INTRODUCTION

Pregnancy represents an intricate physiologic process involving hormonal intercommunication between the maternal brain and developing fetal–placental unit the disequilibrium of which imparts risk of conditions (eg, preeclampsia) that increase morbidity and mortality of the mother–baby dyad. In this chapter, the authors highlight the two most common endocrine disorders in pregnancy, diabetes mellitus (DM) and thyroid disease.

Also highlighted will be the role played by social determinant of health (SDoH) in amplifying pregnancy risk. SDoHs (ie, economic stability, education access and quality, health care access and quality, neighborhood and build environment, and social and community context) are drivers of health outcomes representing almost 80% of

[a] Department of Family and Community Medicine, Penn State College of Medicine, 500 University Drive, HP11, Hershey, PA 17033, USA; [b] Department of Family Medicine, Tidelands Health Medical University of South Carolina Residency Program, 4320 Holmestown Road, Myrtle Beach, SC 29588, USA
* Corresponding author.
E-mail address: sramirez2@pennstatehealth.psu.edu

Prim Care Clin Office Pract 51 (2024) 535–547
https://doi.org/10.1016/j.pop.2024.04.009
0095-4543/24/© 2024 Elsevier Inc. All rights reserved.

the factors directly impacting health.[1,2] Deeply rooted in racism, discrimination, historical insults, and SDoH, the United States has the highest number of pregnancy-related deaths in the developed world. Black maternal care disparities in the United States continue to worsen highlighted by pregnancy-related death being triple the rates of their White counterparts.[2] An understanding of SDoH can serve as a vehicle to empowering prenatal care providers in delivering culturally responsive care thereby helping narrow health disparities for vulnerable populations.

HYPOTHALAMIC–PITUITARY–OVARIAN AXIS

The hormonal feedback mechanisms of the hypothalamic–pituitary–ovarian (HPO) axis are integral to regulating female reproduction. The secretion of gonadotropin-releasing hormone (GnRH) by the hypothalamus on the anterior pituitary gland produces luteinizing hormone (LH) and follicle-stimulating hormone (FSH).[3] LH and FSH, in turn, act on the ovaries to synthesize the sex hormones, estrogen and progesterone, which play critical roles in the proliferative, ovulatory, secretory, and menstruation phases of the menstrual cycle and together trigger a dynamic hormonal cascade in pregnancy, lactation, and post-partum.[3]

THE PLACENTA

The placenta is a novel and highly complex, yet temporary, endocrine organ. It facilitates the exchange of oxygen and carbon dioxide, the synthesis and transfer of nutrients, and the elimination of fetal waste products (eg, urea, creatinine, uric acid). The placenta plays a vital role in maternal–fetal physiology and lactation postpartum. It serves as a physical and immunologic barrier, a hematologic reserve, and manufactures peptides and steroid hormones.[4]

Placental development commences at conception. After an egg becomes fertilized, the developing zygote travels from the fallopian tube to the intrauterine cavity where it develops into a blastocyst. The blastocyst implants into the decidua (endometrium of pregnancy) around day 7 of pregnancy through the actions of chemokines, cytokines, proteolytic enzymes, prostaglandins, and other cellular mediators. The trophoblastic (outer) layer of the blastocyst develops into the maternal side of the placenta, then further differentiates into the inner and fetal aspects of the placenta by week 4.[5]

While the maternal placental circulatory system begins to develop between weeks 1 and 2, fetal development occurs within a low-oxygen environment (Pao$_2$ < 15 mm Hg) until about 10 weeks which serves to protect the fetus from reactive oxygen species during organogenesis.[6,7] Between 10 and 12 weeks, the maternal–placental circulatory system begins transitioning from a low to high oxygen environment in response to arterial remodeling efforts whereby spiral artery caliber increases resulting in straighter flow path decreased resistance.[7] During this time, the proliferative processes within the maternal vessels and villi of the placenta as well as the development of secure connections between the placental villi and fetal vasculature associated with the umbilical cord take place.[7] By 14 weeks the development of the maternal placental circulation is complete. The placenta continues growing with the fetus throughout pregnancy and by term can process a total blood flow rate of approximately 700 mL/minute.[6]

MATERNAL METABOLISM AND FETAL GROWTH REGULATION

Steroid and peptide-based hormones are secreted by the placenta and other neuroendocrine organs inducing adaptations in maternal physiology accommodating fetal growth and development and enabling lactation postpartum. Notable functions of these placental hormones include the regulation of the reproductive axis, maternal metabolism, fetal growth, vasculogenesis, angiogenesis, and stress responses.[8]

During the prenatal period, most placental hormones are synthesized by syncytiotrophoblasts and/or cytotrophoblasts, specialized cells derived from early blastocystic tissue. Growth factors and remaining placental hormones are produced by villous stromal cells and macrophages.[8] Altogether, the regulation of the reproductive axis involves a delicate interplay between these factors and hormones.

- *Beta-subunit of the human chorionic gonadotropin (β-hCG),* a peptide hormone is one of the first hormones secreted by the placenta and, therefore, serves as a clinical marker to diagnose pregnancy. It acts on the corpus luteum to increase progesterone production in the first trimester and also stimulates thyroxine production within the thyroid gland in a manner similar to thyroid-stimulating hormone (TSH).[8] β-hCG production and concentration gradually declines after week 12.
- *Progesterone* is a steroid hormone, and its production is dependent on maternal cholesterol stores. It acts to suppress menstruation throughout pregnancy, prevents premature uterine contractions, prevents feto-placental allograft rejection, and promotes lactogenesis.[8]
- *Estrogen* is a steroid hormone, and its production is dependent on maternal and fetal production of its precursor, dehydroepiandrosterone-sulfate (DHEA-S). Estrogen upregulates protein synthesis required for steroid metabolism and persistent progesterone production. It also maintains adequate uterine blood flow and primes breast tissue for lactation.[8]
- *Corticotropin-releasing hormone, adrenocorticotropin (ACTH),* and *urocortin* are peptide hormones that increase cortisol and prostaglandin production and help trigger fetal DHEA-S secretion.[8]
- *Oxytocin* is a peptide hormone that slowly increases in concentration during pregnancy and peaks at labor onset to promote myometrial contractions.[8]
- *Human placental lactogen (hPL)* is a peptide hormone that works in conjunction with progesterone and prolactin to increase maternal food intake. The increased calories promote maternal weight gain for nutrient storage and later mobilization for fetal and placental growth. Additionally, hPL increases circulating insulin concentration and activity and promotes breast development, lactogenesis, and calcium absorption.[8]
- *Human placental growth hormone (hPGH)* is a peptide hormone that is continuously secreted at increasing concentrations throughout pregnancy. It is involved in fetal and placental growth, lipolysis, and lactogenesis. hPGH is a primary determinant of maternal insulin resistance and gestational diabetes.[8]
- *Prolactin* is a peptide hormone that helps enable blastocyst implantation, triggers maternal hyperphagia, and promotes fetal growth and lactogenesis.[8]
- *Vascular endothelial growth factor (VEGF)* is a family of peptide hormones integral to vasculogenesis early in pregnancy and angiogenesis later in pregnancy. VEGF synthesis is upregulated by hypoxia, and its dysregulation is theorized to be associated with the development of preeclampsia and intrauterine growth restriction.[8]

LACTOGENESIS AND LACTATION

Following delivery, many neuroendocrine responses become hormonally activated promoting lactation, lactational amenorrhea, and restoration of maternal pre-pregnancy physiology. Mammary gland growth induced by hPL, hPGH, and prolactin during pregnancy prepares maternal alveoli for lactation postpartum. As the concentrations of progesterone and estrogen decrease after delivery, their ability to prevent lactogenesis wanes, and lactogenesis ensues in the context of a persistently elevated prolactin level.

Infant suckling involves a neuroendocrine reflex loop. Suckling stimulates the release of prolactin and oxytocin from the anterior pituitary gland that promotes further breast feeding. The prolactin stimulates an increase in milk production, and the release of milk from mammary glands occurs through an oxytocin-triggered myoepithelial cell contractions. Furthermore, lactation inhibits GnRH activity in the hypothalamus, resulting in anovulation which may last up to 6 months postpartum in patients exclusively breastfeeding.[3]

HYPERGLYCEMIC CONDITIONS IN PREGNANCY

As a primary determinant of maternal insulin resistance, hPGH increases the risk of gestational DM.[8] DM imparts significant morbidity to the mother–baby dyad including increased risk of miscarriage, preterm delivery (<37 weeks), preeclampsia, shoulder dystocia, cesarean deliveries, congenital malformations, macrosomia, and admission to the neonatal intensive care unit.[9] Risk factors for insulin resistance and subsequent DM include maternal age 35 years or more, polycystic ovarian syndrome, HIV, metabolic syndrome, prepregnancy body mass index 25 or greater, family history: DM in first degree relative, sedentary lifestyle, hypertension, impaired fasting glucose or prediabetes, history of gestational diabetes, acanthosis nigricans, certain medication use (steroids, antipsychotics, etc.), history of cardiovascular disease, and ethnicity/race (Native American, African American, Latino, Asian American, Pacific Islander).[9] Screening tests for individuals at increased risk of insulin resistance include a hemoglobin A1c, fasting glucose, or 2 h oral glucose tolerance test (OGTT) at the first prenatal visit.[10] Treatment goals should not only include achieving euglycemia through medications but also address the SDoH that may be impeding the patient from adopting a healthy lifestyle.

Insulin Resistance

Pregnancy is characterized by an increased risk of insulin resistance due to placental-produced hormones (ie, human placenta lactogen, progesterone, prolactin, placental growth hormone [GH], cortisol) that increase throughout pregnancy and are greatest in the third trimester.[10] The one exception to these hyperglycemic changes is during late first trimester when elevated levels of estrogen increase insulin sensitivity thereby increasing the risk of maternal hypoglycemia.[10]

Pregestational Diabetes Mellitus

The diagnosis of pregestational DM is made if DM is diagnosed at or before 24 weeks gestation.[10] Pregestational DM commonly includes type 1 (DMI) and type 2 (DMII) which complicate up to 2% of pregnancies in the United States with DMII accounting for up to half of these cases.[9] While the pathophysiology of DMI and DMII is similar, DMI is associated with autoimmunity to the pancreatic beta cells, whereas DMII is primarily a result of peripheral insulin resistance, relative insulin deficiency, and obesity.[10] The diagnosis of DM is made by a hemoglobin A1c greater than 6.4, fasting plasma glucose greater than 125 mg/dL, a random plasma glucose greater than 199 mg/dL, and/or an abnormal OGTT (Table 1).[11,12]

Table 1
Types of oral glucose tolerance tests (OGTT) for the diagnosis of diabetes mellitus[12]

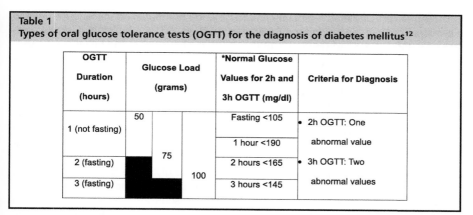

OGTT Duration (hours)	Glucose Load (grams)	*Normal Glucose Values for 2h and 3h OGTT (mg/dl)	Criteria for Diagnosis
1 (not fasting)	50	Fasting <105	• 2h OGTT: One abnormal value
		1 hour <190	
2 (fasting)	75	2 hours <165	• 3h OGTT: Two abnormal values
3 (fasting)	100	3 hours <145	

* Except for the fasting timepoint, all other timepoints are noted as glucose values measured after ingestion of the indicated glucose load. Abnormal value cut offs represent the National Diabetes Data Group criteria.

Diabetic ketoacidosis

Diabetic ketoacidosis (DKA) is a life-threatening emergency in 5% to 10% of all pregnancies complicated by pregestational DM, although it is more common in DMI.[10] DKA can occur in the absence of hyperglycemia (euglycemic ketoacidosis) and should be considered in pregnant individuals with pregestational DM and persistent nausea and vomiting.[9] DKA is marked by arterial acidosis, serum bicarbonate less than 15 mEq/L, elevated anion gap, and the presence of serum ketones.[10]

Due to a high perinatal mortality rate that can reach up to 30% or higher in severe DKA, maternal–fetal status and response to treatment should be closely monitored.[13] Treatment should be done in consultation with maternal–fetal medicine, endocrinology, and anesthesiology. The principles of DKA treatment in pregnancy are similar to nonpregnant populations and included fluid resuscitation, intravenous insulin therapy with the addition of glucose depending on glucose levels, correction of acidosis, treatment of precipitating conditions, and correction of electrolytes.[13] The decision for delivery is challenging and is best made in consultation with other specialists. Delivery is not indicated as treatment for DKA, but may be necessary once maternal stability is obtained and depends on gestational age and maternal–fetal response to treatment.[13]

Gestational Diabetes Mellitus

Gestational DM (GDM) affects 1 in 11 pregnancies in the United States, this is nearly doubled from 2006 to 2017.[14] Screening for GDM at 24 to 28 weeks gestation with a 1 h OGTT is recommended, and if abnormal followed by a 3 h OGTT (**Table 1**).[14] GDM is considered Class A1 (A1GDM) if nutrition alone achieves euglycemia and Class A2 (A2GDM) if medication is required.[14]

Outpatient Management of Diabetes Mellitus

The mainstay of DM treatment includes lifestyle modifications (ie, healthy nutrition, exercise) and glucose monitoring. Studies show that patients using continuous glucose monitoring (CGM) have lower rates of preeclampsia and their neonates have lower rates of hypoglycemia, macrosomia, and NICU admissions.[10] Patients with lower economic status and who are uninsured will be less likely to afford a CGM thereby increasing their risks of worse DM control and more DM-related complications.[15]

The American Diabetes Association recommends nutritional counseling to develop a personalized nutrition plan by a registered dietitian.[12] The recommended diet consists of calories from carbohydrates (33%–40%), protein (20%), and fat (40%)[12]; moderate intensity, aerobic, exercise 30 minutes per day, at least 5 times per week is recommended.[12]

Insulin is preferred as standard therapy in the management of pregestational DM and A2GDM.[12] Insulin dosing should be titrated to achieve a fasting plasma glucose less than 95 (mg/dL), 1 hour postprandial plasma glucose less than 140 (mg/dL), and 2 hour postprandial plasma glucose less than 120 (mg/dL). Typical starting insulin doses in the first trimester include 0.7 to 0.8 units/kg/day, 0.8 to 1 unit/kg/day in the second trimester, and 0.9 to 1.2 units/kg/day in the third trimester.[10]

Noninsulin treatment options include metformin and glyburide. These medications, however, do cross the placenta and the adverse effect on the fetus is unknown. Shared decision making should be included when discussing these medication with patients.[9] Metformin is often considered in pregnant individuals who decline insulin, are unsafe to self-administer insulin, or cannot afford insulin.[12] The starting dose of metformin is 500 mg/day with a max dose of 2500 to 3000 mg/day.[12] Glyburide should rarely, if ever, be used as it is associated with an increased risk of macrosomia, hypoglycemia, preeclampsia, hyperbilirubinemia, and stillbirths compared to insulin.[12]

Uncontrolled hyperglycemia is associated with increased morbidity including microvascular complications (ie, retinopathy, nephropathy); an ophthalmic examination is recommended in the preconception period, during the first trimester, in the second and third trimesters as needed, and within 1 year postpartum based on degree of retinopathy.[9] DM nephropathy may worsen in the prenatal period and monitoring of proteinuria is recommended during this time.

Additionally, pregestational and GDM increase the risk of preeclampsia. Therefore, blood pressure monitoring at each prenatal visit is advised, as well as educating patients on the warning signs of preeclampsia. Screening for nephropathy by way of a spot urine protein/creatine should be done in each trimester and 81 mg to 160 mg/day of aspirin should be started at 12 weeks gestation as preeclampsia prophylaxis.[16]

Fetal surveillance and delivery timing

Determination of the optimal frequency of fetal surveillance and delivery timing should be made in consultation with perinatology. ACOG recommends weekly to biweekly antenatal testing starting at 32 weeks gestation based on glycemic control.[17] Hyperglycemia increases the risk of fetal cardiac anomalies, the most common of which being hypertrophic cardiomyopathy.[18] While most anomalies can be detected at 18 to 20 weeks gestation with an anatomy ultrasound, fetal echocardiogram is recommended in pregnancies complicated by DM.[10] Given the increased risk of fetal macrosomia and its associated morbidity, assessment of fetal growth velocity with ultrasound may be considered.[10]

Delivery timing is based on balancing the risk of fetal death with risks of preterm birth. Delivery between 36 0/7 weeks and 38 6/7 is considered for those with DM complicated by vascular pathology, neuropathy, or hyperglycemia.[19] Consideration may be given for cesarean section in pregnancies complicated by DM and fetal macrosomia (>4500 g) as prophylaxis against traumatic birth injury to the fetus.[20]

Labor Considerations

The use of antenatal steroids for fetal lung maturity increases the risk for increased maternal insulin requirement in the following 5 days and should be discussed with the patient.[10] To prevent fetal and neonatal hyperglycemia, the intrapartum glycemic goal less than or equal to 110 mg/dL should be used.[10] Following delivery, maternal insulin requirements decrease by 33% to 50% of predelivery levels thus continued monitoring of glycemic levels are imperative to assess the need for insulin treatment.[10] For pregnant individuals on insulin pumps insulin doses should be reduced by approximately 50%, to avoid hypoglycemic episodes.[10] Patients with GDM may not require insulin therapy following delivery.

Postpartum Considerations

Approximately half of individuals with GDM will develop DMII within 5 to 10 years post-delivery.[9] GDM also increases the risk of developing GDM earlier in subsequent pregnancies.[14] Screening for DMII in the 4 to 12 weeks postpartum period is recommended with a 2 h OGTT (Table X), and if negative then every 3 years for 10 years with a hemoglobin A1c is recommended.[14]

Breastfeeding is recommended in pregestational DM and GDM and education should include increasing maternal daily caloric intake by 500 calories to avoid hypoglycemia.[10] Close monitoring of glycemic control is encouraged as insulin requirements may decrease by up to 20% due to the discontinuation of placental hormone production.[9]

THYROID DISORDERS DURING PREGNANCY

There is no evidence that screening for thyroid disorders improves pregnancy outcomes. However, because it is the second most common endocrine disorder in pregnancy, providers should be alert for signs and symptoms of thyroid disease (**Table 2**). Without diagnosis and treatment, thyroid disorders can have devastating consequences for both the mother and fetus.

Table 2
Symptoms, signs, and fetal consequences of thyroid disorders in pregnancy[23,27,28]

Maternal Condition	Symptoms	Signs	Fetal Consequences
Hypothyroidism	Cognitive impairment, constipation, depression, difficulty focusing, dry skin, fatigue, hoarseness, coarse fascies, lateral eyebrow thinning, macroglossia, hair changes, arthralgias, infertility, myalgias, weight gain, infertility, menorrhagia	Bradycardia, hyporeflexia, diastolic hypertension, edema, goiter, hypothermia, hoarseness, blood dyscrasias (normocytic anemia, hyperlipidemia, hypertriglyceridemia, hyperprolactinemia, hyponatremia), proteinuria, pericardial effusion, periorbital edema, low voltage electrocardiogram.	Low birth weight, impaired neuro-psychological development, stillbirth. Abruptio placentae, preeclampsia
Hyperthyroidism	Palpitations, anxiety, tremors, frequent stools, hyperhidrosis, intolerance to heat, weight loss, insomnia, photophobia, eye sensitivity, increased lacrimation, diplopia, blurry vision, reduced color perception	Tachycardia, goiter, arrhythmia, edema, orthopnea, hyperpigmentation, hyperreflexia, hypertension, lid lag, lid retraction, pretibial myxedema, periorbital edema, exophthalmos	Miscarriage, preterm birth, low birth weight, stillbirth, tachycardia, thyrotoxicosis

Multiple thyroid-related changes occur in pregnancy. By approximately 12 weeks gestation, the size of the maternal thyroid gland increased due to increased circulation and blood volume.[21] The fetus concentrates iodine thereby increasing iodine requirement by approximately 50%.[21] Additionally, the production of thyroid hormones thyroxine (T4) and triiodothyronine (T3) increases by approximately 50%.[21] The increase concentrations of maternal estrogen results in increased concentrations of thyroid-binding globulin.[22] Altogether resulting in an increase in TSH. During the first 12 weeks of pregnancy, high concentrations of hCG results in weak stimulation of TSH that stimulates secretion of thyroid hormone increasing free T4 (fT4).[23] The elevated fT4 levels cause suppression of TSH-releasing hormone at the level of the hypothalamus which decreases TSH.[23] The fetus is fully reliant on maternal transfer of T4 as its thyroid gland does not become fully functional until 18 to 20 weeks gestation and maternal T4 deficiency negatively impacts fetal brain development.[24] While TSH levels can mirror those in the nonpregnant individual by the second trimester, the levels of T4 and T3 increase due to increases in thyroid-binding globulin.[21]

The identification and management of preexisting thyroid disease in the preconception period allows for optimization of the condition and improved pregnancy outcomes. Similarly, careful history and physical examination to elucidate signs and symptoms of thyroid dysfunction are imperative (see **Table 2**). Should clinical suspicion arise, TSH levels should be measured and if abnormal an fT4 test helps determine the etiology.[25] Given the risks to the developing fetus in pregnancies complicated by poorly controlled thyroid disease, determination of the frequency of antenatal surveillance and timing of delivery should be made in consultation with perinatology.[26] The impact of subclinical hypothyroidism on neurocognitive development of the neonate, on the other hand, is not well understood and the effectiveness of levothyroxine therapy has not been demonstrated.[23]

When evaluating a possible thyroid disorder, it is critical to distinguish whether hyperthyroidism or hypothyroidism is due to abnormal functioning of the thyroid gland (primary) or from dysfunction of the pituitary–hypothalamic axis (central). Primary hypothyroidism is characterized by low fT4 and elevated TSH levels, while central hypothyroidism is characterized by low fT4 and low, normal, or slightly increased TSH levels.[21–23] Primary hyperthyroidism is characterized by an elevated fT4 and low TSH levels, while central hyperthyroidism is characterized by an elevated fT4 and elevated TSH levels.[21–23] Since central thyroid disorders are much less common, this chapter focuses on primary thyroid disorders.

Hypothyroidism

Hypothyroidism complicates 1 to 3 per 1000 pregnancies in the United States and contributes to significant morbidity to the pregnant individual and fetus (**Table 3**).[25]

Diagnostic considerations

Primary hypothyroidism is diagnosed when fT4 is low in the presence of high TSH (see **Table 3**). In iodine sufficient countries, the most common cause of hypothyroidism is Hashimoto thyroiditis.

Outpatient management

Management of primary hypothyroidism in pregnancy should aim to keep the TSH level between the lower limit of the reference range and 2.5 milliunits/L.[23] The first line of treatment for hypothyroidism is levothyroxine and TSH levels should be checked every 4 weeks while levothyroxine doses are being titrated.[23] For individuals with pregestational hypothyroidism, the levothyroxine dose should be increased by an

Table 3
Diagnostic criteria for primary hypothyroidism and hyperthyroidism[3]

Maternal Condition		TSH Level	fT4	Other
Primary Hypothyroidism	Overt	Elevated	Low	
	Subclinical	Elevated	Normal	Elevated thyroid peroxidase antibody[a]
	Hashimoto's	Elevated	Low	Elevated thyroid peroxidase antibody[a]
Primary Hyperthyroidism	Overt	Low	elevated	
	Subclinical	Low	normal	
	Graves	Low	elevated	Elevated stimulating TSH receptor antibodies (TRab)[b]

[a] It is unnecessary to measure thyroid peroxidase antibody to diagnose hypothyroidism but is useful in assessing the risk of progression to overt hypothyroidism in subclinical hypothyroidism.[29].
[b] TRabs are over 90% sensitive and specific in the diagnosis of Graves disease. Baseline TRab assessment should be obtained prior to initiating treatment in pregnant individuals.[30].

extra dose 2 days a week for a total of 9 doses per week in the first trimester with adjustments made based on TSH levels at the first prenatal visit and every 4 weeks thereafter.[21,31] There is a lack of evidence to support the use of T3 in the management of hypothyroidism and in iodine-rich countries the use of iodine supplementation including iodine rich foods does not improve outcomes.[23]

Hyperthyroidism

Hyperthyroidism complicates approximately 1% of pregnancies with Graves disease accounting for 95% of cases.[32] If left untreated, hyperthyroidism can result in preeclampsia with severe features, maternal heart failure, and thyroid storm an acute, life-threatening condition with an estimated mortality up to 25%.[33] As the most common cause of hyperthyroidism, Graves disease is an autoimmune process whereby antibodies stimulate the TSH receptor resulting in excess thyroid hormone production. In the fetus, maternal thyroid-stimulating immunoglobulin and TSH-binding inhibitory immunoglobulins cross the placenta and can result in neonatal hypothyroidism or hyperthyroidism with up to 5% of neonates having Graves disease.[34]

Diagnostic considerations
Primary hyperthyroidism is marked by and elevated fT4 in the setting of a low TSH.

Outpatient management
During the first trimester, preference is given to propylthiouracil (PTU) in the treatment of hyperthyroidism due to the teratogenic risk of methimazole (eg, esophageal or choanal atresia, aplasia cutis).[23] While PTU or methimazole may be used in the second and the third trimesters, methimazole is preferred given the risk of hepatotoxicity with PTU.[23] Serial complete blood counts are not recommended during treatment unless the patient becomes febrile or develops a sore throat at which time treatment should be discontinued and screening for agranulocytosis undertaken.[23] Monitoring fT4 every 4 weeks during treatment is recommended with a goal fT4 at or slightly above reference range.[21]

The initiation of PTU in the first trimester is based on severity of illness and oral dosage ranges between 100 mg and 600 mg divided into 3 doses daily with typical doses ranging between 200 mg and 400 mg.[21] PTU is discontinued and Methimazole started int he second trimester. Methimazole is started at doses between 5 mg and 30 mg divided into 2 doses transitioning to once daily dosing during the maintenance phase.[21] Should transition between PTU and Methimazole be required, this is achieved using a 20:1 conversion.[23] Adjunct therapy with oral propranolol (10 mg to 40 mg 3 to 4 times daily) in the setting of palpitations is recommended until a euthyroid state is reached.[21]

Postpartum Thyroiditis

Thyroid dysfunction within the first 12 months after delivery is diagnostic of postpartum thyroiditis which may present with symptoms and signs of hypothyroidism, hyperthyroidism, or both. The pathogenesis of postpartum thyroiditis involves destruction of the thyroid gland within the first 4 months postpartum leading to excessive release of thyroid hormone and decreased TSH followed by decreased levels of thyroid hormone and overt hypothyroidism 4 to 8 months postpartum. While PTU and methimazole are ineffective in halting this process, beta blockers may be helpful in the symptomatic patient. In approximately 30% of patients, hypothyroidism persists necessitating treatment with levothyroxine therefore periodic thyroid testing is recommended.[23]

OTHER PREGNANCY-RELATED ENDOCRINE CONDITIONS

Other endocrine conditions that providers should be aware of when treating pregnant patients include Sheehan syndrome and prolactinoma. Regarding these conditions, this article will briefly review key concepts for providers to be aware.

Sheehan Syndrome

Sheehan Syndrome is a rare pregnancy-related condition causing deficiency of pituitary hormones due to postpartum ischemic injury of the anterior pituitary gland from blood loss and hypovolemia. Prolactin and GH are the most common hormones affected. GH is impacted first with Sheehan syndrome followed by prolactin, FSH, LH, ACTH, and finally TSH.[35] The signs and symptoms of Sheehan syndrome may not present until weeks or months after delivery with agalactorrhea the most common symptom, but other symptoms include amenorrhea or oligomenorrhea, hot flashes, decreased sex drive, fatigue, bradycardia, hypotension, cold intolerance, weight gain, weight loss, constipation, and loss of axillary and pubic hair.[35] The acute postpartum hypotension and tachycardia of adrenal dysfunction in Sheehan syndrome can be confused with hypovolemia and shock. Hyponatremia and persistent hypoglycemia can help differentiate Sheehan syndrome from other causes of hypotension.[35] MRI evaluation of the pituitary can confirm the diagnosis and patients should be referred to endocrinology for treatment that includes correcting hormone deficiencies.

Prolactinoma

Prolactinomas are the most prevalent functional benign pituitary tumors. Because it causes infertility and gonadal dysfunction, it is rare for patients with functional prolactinomas to become pregnant. Managing prolactinomas during pregnancy can be challenging because the hyperestrogen state of pregnancy may increase the tumor volume with potential mass effects.[36] Because of the complexity of prolactinoma during pregnancy, treatment should involve multiple specialists including perinatology, endocrinology, and neurosurgery.

DISCUSSION

Pregnancy is a unique endocrine process. This chapter was not intended to address every endocrine condition encountered in pregnancy, but rather focused on the most common: hyperglycemic diseases and thyroid disorders. These conditions affect both fetal and maternal health and increase the risk of morbidity and mortality. The authors reviewed how SDoH can affect these risks and outcomes of patients.

SUMMARY

Pregnancy is a highly sophisticated and specialized neuroendocrine mechanism governed by the maternal HPO axis in promoting placental development and fetal growth, a process aided by protein and steroid hormones in conjunction with cell-signaling molecules. Dysregulation in placental VEGF, hPGH, maternal glucose metabolism, and thyroid function imparts increased morbidity and mortality to the pregnancy and developing fetus including but not limited to DM, thyroid dysfunction, and preeclampsia. It is therefore recommended to screen for these conditions in pregnant individuals at high risk and consider the impact SDoH play on perpetuating this risk.

CLINICS CARE POINTS

- Pregnant individuals at risk of preeclampsia, including those diagnosed with DM, should be started on prophylactic daily low-dose aspirin (81 mg) between 12 and 16 weeks gestation.
- Options for screening individuals at increased risk of insulin resistance (see **Table 1**) include a hemoglobin A1c, fasting glucose, or 2-h oral glucose tolerance test at the first prenatal visit.
- Individuals with DM should be encouraged to adopt a healthy lifestyle including a diet consisting of calories from carbohydrates (33% to 40%), protein (20%), and fat (40%) as well as moderate intensity, aerobic, exercise 30 minutes/day, at least 5 times/week.
- While there is no evidence that screening for thyroid disorders improves pregnancy outcomes, a TSH should be checked in individuals with signs or symptoms of thyroid dysfunction.

DISCLOSURE

The authors have no relevant disclosures.

REFERENCES

1. Robert Wood Johnson Foundation. Going beyond clinical walls: solving complex problems. Institute for Clinical Systems Improvement. 2014. Available at: https://www.icsi.org/wp-content/uploads/2019/08/1.SolvingComplexProblems_BeyondClinicalWalls.pdf. [Accessed 12 November 2023].
2. Hoyert DL. Maternal mortality rates in the United States, 2021. NCHS Health E-Stats 2023. https://doi.org/10.15620/cdc:113967.
3. Xu C, Papadakis G, Pitteloud N. Normal endocrine physiology of hypothalamic hormones during ovulation, pregnancy, and lactation. In: Kovacs C, Deal C, editors. Maternal-fetal and neonatal endocrinology: physiology, pathophysiology, and clinical management. 1st edition; 2020. p. 7–14.
4. Wright C, Sibley C. Placental transfer in health and disease. In: Kay H, Nelson M, Wang Y, editors. The placenta: from development to disease. First. Blackwell Publishing Ltd; 2011. p. 66–74. https://doi.org/10.1002/9781444393927.
5. Aplin J, Kimber S. Trophoblast-uterine interactions at implantation. Reprod Biol Endocrinol 2004;2(48). https://doi.org/10.1186/1477-7827-2-48. . [Accessed 12 November 2023].

6. Cunningham F, Leveno K, Bloom S, et al. Embryogenesis and fetal morphological developments. In: Williams obstetrics. 25th edition. McGraw Hill Education; 2018. p. 124–43.

7. Rampersad R, Cervar-Zivkovic M, Nelson M. Development and anatomy of the human placenta. In: Kay H, Nelson M, Wang Y, editors. The placenta: from development to disease. 1st edition. Blackwell Publishing Ltd; 2011. p. 17–26.

8. McNamara J, Kay H. Placental hormones: physiology, disease, and prenatal diagnosis. In: Kay H, Nelson D, Wang Y, editors. The placenta: from development to disease. 1st edition. Blackwell Publishing Ltd; 2011. p. 57–65.

9. Raets L, Ingelbrecht A, Benhalima K. Management of type 2 diabetes in pregnancy: a narrative review. Front Endocrinol 2023;14.

10. American College of Obstetricians and Gynecologists' Committee on Practice Bulletins-Obstetrics. Pregestational Diabetes Mellitus: ACOG Practice Bulletin, Number 201. Obstet Gynecol 2018;132(6):e228–48.

11. Diagnosis | ADA. Available at: https://diabetes.org/about-diabetes/diagnosis. [Accessed 19 November 2023].

12. Caughey AB, Turrentine M. Gestational diabetes mellitus: ACOG Practice Bulletin, Number 190. Obstet Gynecol 2018;131(2):e49–64.

13. Sibai BM, Viteri OA. Diabetic ketoacidosis in pregnancy. Obstet Gynecol 2014; 123(1):167–78.

14. Will JS, Crellin H. Gestational diabetes mellitus: update on screening, diagnosis, and management. Am Fam Physician 2023;108(3):249–58. Available at: https:// www.aafp.org/pubs/afp/issues/2023/0900/gestational-diabetes.html. [Accessed 12 November 2023].

15. Blonde L, Umpierrez GE, Reddy SS, et al. American Association of Clinical Endocrinology Clinical Practice Guideline: Developing a Diabetes Mellitus Comprehensive Care Plan—2022 Update. Endocr Pract 2022;28(10).

16. Davidson KW, Barry MJ, Mangione CM, et al. Aspirin use to prevent preeclampsia and related morbidity and mortality: us preventive services task force recommendation statement. JAMA 2021;326(12):1186–91.

17. American College of Obstetricians and Gynecologists' Committee on Obstetric Practice, Society for Meternal-Fetal Medicine. Indications for Outpatient Antenatal Fetal Surveillance: ACOG Committee Opinion, Number 828. Obstet Gynecol 2021;137(6):e177–97.

18. Al-Biltagi M, razaky O El, El Amrousy D. Cardiac changes in infants of diabetic mothers. World J Diabetes 2021;12(8):1233.

19. Medically Indicated Late-Preterm and Early-Term Deliveries. ACOG Committee Opinion, Number 831. Obstet Gynecol 2021;138(1):E35–9.

20. Macrosomia: ACOG Practice Bulletin. Number 216. Obstet Gynecol 2020;135(1): E18–35.

21. Alexander EK, Pearce EN, Brent GA, et al. Guidelines of the American Thyroid Association for the diagnosis and management of thyroid disease during pregnancy and the postpartum. Thyroid 2017;27(3):315–89.

22. Visser WE, Peeters RP. Interpretation of thyroid function tests during pregnancy. Best Pract Res Clin Endocrinol Metabol 2020;34(4).

23. American College of Obstetricians and Gynecologists' Committee on Practice Bulletins-Obstetrics. Thyroid disease in pregnancy: ACOG Practice Bulletin, Number 223. Obstet Gynecol 2020;135(6):1496–9.

24. Burrow GN, Fisher DA, Larsen PR. Maternal and fetal thyroid function. N Engl J Med 1994;331(16):1072–8.

25. Ramirez S. Prenatal care: an evidence-based approach. Am Fam Physician 2023;108(2):139–50. Available at: https://pubmed.ncbi.nlm.nih.gov/37590852/. [Accessed 12 November 2023].

26. American College of Obstetricians and Gynecologists' Committee on Practice Bulletins-Obstetrics. Antepartum Fetal Surveillance: ACOG Practice Bulletin, Number 229. Obstet Gynecol 2021;137(6):e116–27.

27. Kravets I. Hyperthyroidism: diagnosis and treatment. Am Fam Physician 2016; 93(5):363–70. Available at: https://www.aafp.org/pubs/afp/issues/2016/0301/p363.html. [Accessed 12 November 2023].

28. Wilson SA, Stem LA, Bruehlman RD. Hypothyroidism: diagnosis and treatment. Am Fam Physician 2021;103(10):605–13. Available at: https://www.aafp.org/pubs/afp/issues/2021/0515/p605.html. [Accessed 12 November 2023].

29. Huber G, Staub JJ, Meier C, et al. Prospective study of the spontaneous course of subclinical hypothyroidism: prognostic value of thyrotropin, thyroid reserve, and thyroid antibodies. J Clin Endocrinol Metab 2002;87(7):3221–6.

30. Barbesino G, Tomer Y. Clinical review: clinical utility of TSH receptor antibodies. J Clin Endocrinol Metab 2013;98(6):2247–55.

31. Yassa L, Marqusee E, Fawcett R, et al. Thyroid hormone early adjustment in pregnancy (the THERAPY) trial. J Clin Endocrinol Metab 2010;95(7):3234–41.

32. Dong AC, Stagnaro-Green A. Differences in diagnostic criteria mask the true prevalence of thyroid disease in pregnancy: a systematic review and meta-analysis. Thyroid 2019;29(2):278–89.

33. Pokhrel B, Aiman W, Bhusal K. Thyroid Storm. StatPearls 2022. Available at: https://www.ncbi.nlm.nih.gov/books/NBK448095/. [Accessed 19 November 2023].

34. Van Der Kaay DCM, Wasserman JD, Palmert MR. Management of neonates born to mothers with Graves' disease. Pediatrics 2016;137(4).

35. Karaca Z, Laway BA, Dokmetas HS, et al. Sheehan syndrome. Nat Rev Dis Prim 2016;2:16092.

36. Almalki MH, Alzahrani S, Alshahrani F, et al. Managing Prolactinomas during Pregnancy. Front Endocrinol 2015;6:85.

Neuroendocrine Neoplasms

Sukhjeet Kamboj, MD[a], Francis Guerra-Bauman, MD[a],
Hussain Mahmud, MD[b], Abdul Waheed, MD, MS PHS, CPE[c],*

KEYWORDS

- Neuroendocrine neoplasms (NENs) • Neuroendocrine tumors (NETs) • Carcinoid
- Incidentaloma • Adrenal tumors • Merkel cell tumor • Pheochromocytoma
- Gastropancreatic

KEY POINTS

- Neuroendocrine neoplasms (NENs), also known as neuroendocrine tumors (NETs), are a group of highly heterogeneous tumors originating from neuroendocrine cells.
- A vast majority of NETs remain asymptomatic and are detected incidentally.
- Carcinoid crisis is an acute life-threatening presentation of carcinoid syndrome characterized by profound flushing, bronchospasm, and rapidly fluctuating blood pressure.
- An insulinoma is a pancreatic NEN that produces insulin and can present with symptoms of hypoglycemia that include tachycardia, fatigue, tremors, shakiness, diaphoresis, confusion, and seizures.
- Pheochromocytoma is a rare adrenal NEN that can present with hypertension, palpitations, sweating, headache, and hyperglycemia.
- Merkel cell tumors are rare NENs that typically present as firm, painless, nodules on sun-exposed skin and are highly aggressive skin cancers with a high mortality rate.
- Primary care physicians can play a key role in coordinating a multidisciplinary team of subspecialists in the diagnosis and treatment of NENs.

INTRODUCTION TO NEUROENDOCRINE NEOPLASMS

Neuroendocrine neoplasms (NENs) are rare tumors derived from cells with characteristics of both nerve and endocrine cells and can occur in various organs throughout the body. Cells derived from neuroectoderm migrate to the adrenal glands, various paraganglia, and the olfactory membrane, while those exhibiting epithelial characteristics are predominantly found in the mucosa of the gastrointestinal tract and bronchial system, as well as in the thyroid, the parathyroid glands, and the pancreatic islets.[1]

[a] Department of Family Medicine, WellSpan Good Samaritan Hospital Family Medicine Residency Program, PO Box 1520, Lebanon, PA 17042, USA; [b] Department of Medicine, Endocrinology Fellowship, University of Pittsburgh Medical College, UPMC Center for Endocrinology & Metabolism, 3601 5th Avenue, Falk Suite 3B, Pittsburgh, PA 15213, USA; [c] Department of Family Medicine, Dignity Health Medical Group/Creighton University SOM, Suite 2021, Gilbert, AZ 85297, USA
* Corresponding author.
E-mail address: Abdul.waheed@commonspirit.org

Prim Care Clin Office Pract 51 (2024) 549–560
https://doi.org/10.1016/j.pop.2024.04.010
0095-4543/24/© 2024 Elsevier Inc. All rights reserved.

While NENs universally express markers such as synaptophysin and chromogranin A, they exhibit significant diversity in clinical presentation, functionality, paraneoplastic syndromes (PNSs), histologic features, molecular profile, and prognosis.[1]

Typically diagnosed between the ages of 30 and 50 years, they are more prevalent in women, with an incidence of 4 to 5 cases per 100,000 adults. While appendiceal NENs show stable incidence rates, those in the small intestine, rectum, and stomach are on the rise. Reported incidence rates and survival durations have increased over time, indicating a higher prevalence than previously understood.

NENs can be incidentally discovered during imaging or surgery for unrelated conditions or as part of an evaluation for a specific NEN, based on clinical symptoms. When NENs cause symptoms by secreting hormones, they are called "functioning" tumors. Most NENs do not produce active hormones and are called "nonfunctioning."[1–3] The presentation of neuroendocrine tumors (NETs) varies widely. Common syndromes from functional NENs and their common symptoms are summarized in **Table 1**.

While symptoms of hormone overproduction are characteristic of NETs, only a small number of patients show such symptoms initially.[3] Both functioning and nonfunctioning NENs often present late with vague symptoms that are commonly attributed to other conditions.[4,5] Alternatively, some NENs may present with mass effect symptoms such as gastrointestinal NENs that can cause abdominal discomfort, bowel obstruction, recurrent intussusception. Common symptoms for gastropancreatic and bronchopulmonary NENs are summarized in **Tables 2** and **3**.[2,4]

PARANEOPLASTIC SYNDROMES

PNS is a term used to denote syndromes secondary to substances secreted from NETs not related to their specific organ or tissue of origin and/or production of autoantibodies against tumor cells. These syndromes are mainly associated with hormonal and neurologic symptoms.

Pathophysiology of Common Neuroendocrine Tumor-Related Paraneoplastic Syndromes

- Tumor production and secretion of biologically active hormones leading to endocrine disorders
- Tumor production of cytokines leading to fever, fatigue, weight loss, and cachexia
- Tumor stimulation of antibody formation leading to neurologic manifestations

CARCINOID SYNDROME
Typical Case Presentation

A 50 year old woman comes to the physician due to periodic reddening of her skin that is starting to become bothersome. The redness is mainly on her face and neck and is accompanied by mild warmth. The episodes used to last a couple of minutes, but now they sometimes last over 15 minutes. Lately, she has also had watery diarrhea and some abdominal pain in the last several months. On her examination, she had many vascular purplish spots surrounding her nose. Urinary excretion of 5 hydroxy indole acetic acid (HIAA) was measured in her urine and was increased. CT scan of the abdomen showed a tumor in the small intestine.

Introduction

NETs may rarely present as carcinoid syndrome, which is characterized by flushing, diarrhea, abdominal pain, bronchospasm, telangiectasia, and right-sided heart failure

Table 1
Functional neuroendocrine neoplasms[1–5]

Type/Syndrome	Location	Active Hormone	Clinical Presentation
Carcinoid syndrome	Small intestine, lungs, and pancreas	Serotonin, prostaglandin, tachykinin	• Flushing • Diarrhea • Valvular heart disease • Bronchospasm
Gastrinoma (Zollinger–Ellison)	Pancreas or duodenum	Gastrin	• Peptic ulcer disease, gastroesophageal reflux, burning abdominal pain • Weight loss • Diarrhea, steatorrhea • Can be a part of MEN-1 syndrome
Glucagonoma	Alpha cells of the pancreas	Glucagon	• Hyperglycemia • Necrolytic migratory erythema • Weight loss • May be part of with MEN-1 syndrome
Insulinoma (Whipple triad)	Beta cell of the pancreas	Insulin/proinsulin	• Hypoglycemia • Tachycardia, tremors/shakiness, diaphoresis • Confusion • Seizures.
Somatostatinoma	Neuroendocrine cells of duodenum and pancreas	Somatostatin	• Nonspecific symptoms such as weight loss • Diarrhea/steatorrhea • Diabetes • Gallstones
Vasoactive intestinal, peptide-secreting tumors Verner–Morrison syndrome	Non-beta-cell pancreatic islet cells	Vasoactive intestinal peptide	• Severe watery diarrhea • Hypokalemia • Muscle weakness
Atypical carcinoid syndrome	Foregut	Histamine, 5HTP	• Pruritus • Cutaneous wheals • Bronchospasm
Ectopic Cushing's syndrome	Lungs	ACTH	• Obesity • Facial plethora • Skin atrophy • Easy bruising • Striae • Proximal myopathy • Hyperglycemia

Abbreviations: 5HTP, 5-hydroxy tryptophan; ACTH: adrenocroticotropin hormone.

due to the release of vasoactive substances such as serotonin, histamine, prostaglandins, kallikrein, bradykinins, substance P, and neuron-specific enolase.[2,4] It occurs when hormones produced by NETs reach systemic circulation. Carcinoid syndrome commonly occurs after metastasis to the lungs, but most often occurs after liver metastases develop, allowing for bypass of hepatic metabolism that may inactivate the hormones.

Retrospective cohort studies report that carcinoid syndrome occurs in 6%–13% of patients with pathologically confirmed gastrointestinal NETs and in less than 1% of patients with bronchopulmonary NETs.[6–9] Hindgut tumors (distal colon and rectum) are typically hormonally silent and do not cause carcinoid syndrome.[9]

Evaluation

The workup for diagnosis of NETs includes imaging studies such as CT scans, MRI, and somatostatin receptor scintigraphy for localization and staging. 68-Ga-DOTA-TATE PET-CT scans have gradually replaced octreotide scans as the imaging modality of choice both for diagnostic and staging purposes. Definitive diagnosis requires histopathological examination, including immunohistochemical staining for neuroendocrine markers, measurements of serotonin, chromogranin A in serum, and metabolites such as 5 HIAA in 24 hour urine.

Treatment

For symptomatic relief of acute symptoms, such as diarrhea and bronchospasm, the somatostatin analog octreotide is commonly utilized. Lanreotide is sometimes used off-label to help control symptoms of carcinoid syndrome, as well. Telotristat (Xermelo) can be combined with these drugs to further control diarrhea caused by carcinoid syndrome. Diarrhea associated with carcinoid syndrome can lead to fluid and electrolyte imbalance and/or nutritional deficiencies, necessitating careful monitoring and appropriate interventions.

The primary treatment of localized NETs causing carcinoid syndrome involves surgical removal. For localized tumors, especially in the gastrointestinal tract, surgical resection remains a cornerstone of treatment; increasingly, minimally invasive surgical techniques are being employed for improved patient outcomes.

In cases of metastatic disease, a multidisciplinary team approach that includes collaborating with oncologists, surgeons, and involving endocrinology specialists is ideal. Advanced carcinoid tumors can metastasize, commonly to the liver. Carcinoid heart disease may develop leading to fibrosis of the heart valves and right-sided heart failure. For treatment of metastatic disease, somatostatin analogs provide symptom control and slow tumor growth. Consider targeted therapies, especially in cases of advanced or metastatic disease. It is important to emphasize to patients and caregivers the importance of long-term follow-up for tumor surveillance and managing potential complications.

Complications

Carcinoid crisis is an acute life-threatening presentation of carcinoid syndrome characterized by profound flushing, bronchospasm, and rapidly fluctuating blood pressure. There is little evidence to guide best treatment of, but common treatment includes the use of octreotide, anxiolytics, and antihistamines. It may be precipitated by induction of anesthesia or palpation, ablation, or embolization of an NET, so patients should be given a somatostatin analog before any anesthetic or tumor manipulation.[10–12]

Table 2 Common symptoms with frequency rate in gastropancreatic neuroendocrine neoplasms[2-4]	
Proportion of Patient with Different Symptoms in Gastropancreatic NENs	
Abdominal Pain	28%–79%
Bowel Obstruction	18%–24%
Diarrhea	10%–32%
Carcinoid Heart Disease	8%–19%
Flushing	4%–25%
Gastrointestinal Bleeding	4%–10%
Incidental	9%–18%

GASTROPANCREATIC NEUROENDOCRINE NEOPLASMS
Typical Case Presentation

A 53 year old woman presented with 2 months of watery diarrhea, severe generalized weakness, 7 kg of weight loss, a facial rash, and hypokalemia. A colonoscopy did not reveal the cause of the chronic diarrhea. Biochemical testing showed markedly elevated serum vasoactive intestinal peptide (VIP) and pancreatic polypeptide. A computed tomography (CT) scan of the abdomen and pelvis revealed a 5 cm distal pancreatic mass. Octreoscan showed an intense uptake in the area of the pancreatic mass. Additional biochemical testing revealed a markedly elevated urinary dopamine level.

Introduction

Pancreatic neuroendocrine tumors (PNETs) are rare neoplasms of the pancreas and compose of less than 2% of all pancreatic tumors. These include insulinomas, gastrinomas, glucagonoma, and somatostatinomas. Collectively, these neoplasms are classified as functioning PNETs. Nonfunctioning PNETs are pancreatic tumors with neuroendocrine differentiation but without any clinical syndrome of hormone hypersecretion.[13,14]

PNETs are more common in individuals aged 30 to 60 years, though they can occur at any age. A family history of PNETs or other endocrine tumors may elevate the risk.[13,14]

Symptoms

Most gastropancreatic NETs are nonfunctional and present fairly late with symptoms of mass effects or distant metastases. Clinically, patients can present with symptoms including abdominal pain, weight loss, nausea, and jaundice. Functioning PNETs present specific symptoms, related to the type of hormone they produce. For example,

Table 3 Common symptoms with frequency rate in bronchopulmonary neuroendocrine neoplasms[2-6]	
Proportion of Patient with Different Symptoms in Bronchopulmonary NENs	
Cough	5%–27%
Hemoptysis	23%–32%
Recurrent Infection	41%–49%
Incidentaloma	17%–39%

insulinomas can present with hypoglycemia. Common presenting symptoms of gastropancreatic NETs are summarized in **Table 4**.

Evaluation

Evaluation depends on the specific tumor type and associated symptoms (see **Table 4**), but CT or MRI may help identify and further classify the PNET.

Treatment

The primary approach to treating PNETs involves surgical removal for cases localized within the pancreas and specific patients with metastatic disease. While somatostatin

Table 4
Summary of pancreatic neuroendocrine neoplasms[1–4,7,15]

Type	Location	Active Hormone	Clinical Presentation
Gastrinoma (Zollinger–Ellison)	Pancreas or duodenum	Gastrin	Peptic ulcer disease, gastroesophageal reflux, burning abdominal pain, diarrhea, weight loss, excessive fat in the stool Sometimes it can be a part of MEN-1 syndrome
Glucagonoma	Alpha cells pancreas	Glucagon	Hyperglycemia, severe swelling or irritation of the skin, mouth sores, anemia, weight loss; it could be associated with MEN-1 syndrome
Insulinoma	Beta cell of the pancreas	Insulin	Hypoglycemia which reflective tachycardia, tremors/shakiness, diaphoresis, confusion, and seizures
Somatostatinoma	Neuroendocrine cells of duodenum and pancreas	Somatostatin	Nonspecific symptoms such as weight loss, diarrhea, nausea, vomiting, diabetes, gallstones, weight loss, and steatorrhea
VIPoma Vasoactive intestinal, peptide secreting tumors Verner–Morrison syndrome	Non-beta-cell pancreatic islet cells	Vasoactive intestinal peptide (VIP)	Severe watery, diarrhea, hypokalemia, muscle weakness

analogs have shown considerable efficacy in alleviating symptoms associated with hormone overproduction, the range of available systemic therapies for advanced disease remains constrained. Family physician should take a multidisciplinary approach for diagnosis and management by involving radiology, endocrinology, and surgery early on in the case.[16]

Adrenal Tumors

Adrenal tumors, both functional and nonfunctional, are commonly encountered in primary care. Most adrenal tumors are nonfunctional (75%), benign, and discovered incidentally during imaging for unrelated issues.[17] They occur in 1% to 6% of adults.[17] Functional adrenal adenomas can autonomously overproduce glucocorticoids causing hypercortisolism, mineralocorticoids causing hypertension, and rarely androgens or estrogens, causing virilization or feminization, respectively. **Table 5** summarizes the key adrenal tumors.[17]

Adrenocortical carcinoma (ACC) is rare, accounting for only 2% of adrenal incidentalomas. They are aggressive, carry a poor prognosis, may be functional (hormone secreting), and can occur at any age.[18] The peak incidence is before age 5 years and between 40 and 60 years of age. Family physicians can play a key role in coordinating a multidisciplinary treatment team and carrying out the patient's goals of care.

Certain adrenal disorders may have a gender preference. A family history of adrenal tumors or related syndromes can contribute to an increased risk. Hereditary conditions such as multiple endocrine neoplasia (MEN), von Hippel–Lindau (VHL) syndrome, and familial pheochromocytoma–paraganglioma syndromes increase the risk.[19]

Evaluation

Assessment of adrenal incidentalomas can get convoluted. A well-accepted approach is to start parallel assessment for malignancy and functional status. The functional assessment includes plasma or 24 hour urine collection for metanephrines and catecholamines to evaluate for pheochromocytoma; 8 AM serum cortisol level after 1 mg dexamethasone administration the prior night is performed to assess adrenal hyperfunction and diagnose Cushing's syndrome. Other tests include aldosterone-to-renin ratio (ARR) to investigate primary aldosteronism as elevation of ARR suggests this diagnosis.[17] Radiologic assessment is key in determining whether the incidental finding represents a benign or malignant tumor. Imaging modalities include CT scan with adrenal protocol (precontrast, postcontrast, and 10 minute delayed images) and MRI for characterization of adrenal lesions. Histopathology with tissue sampling may be necessary for definitive diagnosis in certain cases.[17] Early collaboration with radiology for following ACR Appropriateness Criteria and recommendations for interpretation of imaging modalities could work in favor. If it is determined to be benign, close follow-up per ACR recommendations could be instituted by the primary care physician. For cases where functional status comes out to be positive on biochemical testing or malignancy is suspected, an early on multidisciplinary approach with consultations and collaboration with radiology, endocrinology, surgery, and oncology is useful.

A specialized adrenal CT protocol is the preferred imaging method to determine whether an adrenal mass measuring greater than 1 cm but less than 4 cm and greater than 10 Hounsfield units (HU) qualifies as a benign adenoma. An adrenal mass demonstrating diagnostic features of a benign lesion, such as microscopic fat, cyst, or bleeding as evidenced by changes in precontrast and postcontrast imaging less than 10 HU, requires no further workup. Similarly, a calcified mass, such as an old hematoma or calcification from a prior granulomatous infection, does not necessitate additional imaging if the density on an unenhanced CT is less than 10 HU or if there is signal loss compared to the spleen on opposed phase images of a chemical shift MRI. These features invariably indicate a lipid-rich adenoma, irrespective of size, obviating the need for further imaging. Radiologists should review prior imaging examinations whenever possible to assess the stability of the adrenal mass before ordering new imaging studies. Even if the prior imaging studies are not of the same type, previous images containing the adrenal gland, such as chest CT/CT, abdominal ultrasound, or lumbar MRI, can aid in management decisions.[20]

Treatment

When treating patients with adrenal tumors, regular monitoring of blood pressure is warranted. Consider prompt referral to an endocrinologist for hormonal evaluation and surgical consultation for suspicious or functional adrenal lesions. Surgical considerations such as adrenalectomy are indicated for functioning tumors, suspicious lesions, or those with a risk of malignancy; in other instances, laparoscopic adrenalectomy is often preferred for benign adenomas. Important aspects of postoperative care include the need for glucocorticoid replacement after the removal of cortisol-secreting tumors.[17,21] Family physicians can play a key role in coordinating a multidisciplinary treatment team and conducting goals of care discussions early on after and on the way to diagnosis.

PHEOCHROMOCYTOMA
Typical Case Presentation

A 67 year old man was seen by his family physician because of recurrent abdominal pain. An abdominal CT scan was performed, and the patient was noted to have a 3.5 cm large suprarenal nodule. He had a history of anxiety, hypertension, dyslipidemia, obesity, and palpitations, for which he had a cardiology consultation. The patient also reported tremor and a lack of strength in the lower limbs. On physical examination, he had normal abdominal examination without palpable masses and normal heart sounds. Laboratory studies revealed elevated urinary metanephrines and normetanephrine levels.

Introduction

Pheochromocytoma is a rare functional adrenal tumor that results in excess production of epinephrine and/or norepinephrine. They arise from the adrenal medulla, in contrast to adrenal adenomas and ACCs that arise from the adrenal cortex. The incidence of pheochromocytoma is 0.8 per 100,000 person-years.[22] Individuals with a family history of pheochromocytoma or related genetic syndromes are at an increased risk. Pheochromocytomas can be associated with hereditary conditions such as MEN type 2 (MEN2), VHL syndrome, and neurofibromatosis type 1.

Symptoms

About 40% of patients with pheochromocytoma present with the classic triad of hypertension, headache, and diaphoresis.[22] The symptoms are often paroxysmal rather than sustained.[22] Patients can present with hyperadrenergic symptoms such as hypertensive crises with paroxysms of severe hypertension, palpitations, tachycardia, diaphoresis, flushing, headaches, and tremors. Uncommon symptoms include orthostatic hypotension, hyperglycemia, cardiomyopathy, and secondary erythrocytosis. Abdominal pain may occur due to tumor compression or stretching of the adrenal capsule especially with large nonfunctional tumors.[23]

Table 5
Types of adrenal tumors[17]

Location	Type of Tumor	Active Hormone	Clinical Presentation
Adrenal cortex	Adrenocortical adenoma	Nonfunctional	Diagnosed incidentally
Adrenal cortex	Cortisol-producing adenoma	Cortisol	Cushing's syndrome
Adrenal cortex	Mineralocorticoid-secreting adenoma	Aldosterone	Conn's syndrome
Adrenal cortex	Adrenocortical carcinoma	Variable; cortisol, androgens, mineralocorticoids	Variable, depending on hormone being produced.
Adrenal medulla	Pheochromocytoma	Catecholamines	Episodes of hypertension, palpitations, sweating, headache, and hyperglycemia

Evaluation

The evaluation includes plasma or 24 hour urinary metanephrines. Imaging studies include CT/MRI abdomen for localizing the tumor and surgical planning.G-68 PET scan can be considered when metastatic disease is suspected. The pheochromocytoma often is part of the differential diagnosis of hypertensive emergency, urgency, labile hypertension, and other clinical scenarios of difficult to control hypertension, where a concern for secondary hypertension is present. However, clinicians should use careful evaluation of the clinical picture instead of routine ordering of testing to "rule out" pheochromocytoma. Most often, basic metabolic panel along with other clinical data at the time of paroxysmal elevation of blood pressure and other sympathetic hyper-responsive state provides significantly low, intermediate, or high pretest probability. Patients with low to intermediate probability should go only initial basic metabolic profile and electrolyte testing while stabilizing and considering other differential diagnosis higher on the list. However, those with higher pretest probability should under prompt further evaluation with both radiologic and biochemical testing.[24]

Treatment

Laparoscopic surgery is the treatment of choice for pheochromocytoma. Appropriate alpha-adrenergic blockade should be initiated by endocrinologist or endocrine surgeon prior to any intervention, to avoid catecholamine surge-induced acute hypertensive crisis.[25,26] Early expert consultation among cases with high pretest probability could help with prompt diagnosis and management with less further crisis episodes.

MERKEL CELL TUMORS
Introduction

Merkel cell tumors are rare but highly aggressive skin cancers with a high mortality rate.[27] It is more common in older adults, particularly those over the age of 50 years with a median age at diagnosis of 75 to 80 years. The incidence of these NETs has been rising, noted to be more common in certain populations, including Caucasians and males, and more prevalent in individuals with fair skin.[27] Merkel cell tumor carcinogenesis has been associated with chronic exposure to ultraviolet radiation, such as sunlight, and in some cases with the presence of the Merkel cell polyomavirus also known as human polyomavirus5 infection. Immunosuppression is another risk factor as individuals with weakened immune systems, either due to medical conditions or immunosuppressive medications, are at higher risk of developing Merkel cell carcinoid.[27,28]

Clinical Presentation

Merkel cell carcinomas typically present as firm, painless, nodules on the skin. They commonly occur on sun-exposed areas of the skin but can occur in areas not exposed to sunlight. The nodule may be skin-colored or appear in shades of red, blue, or purple. The lesions are generally asymptomatic and can mimic benign lesions or malignancies such as cutaneous squamous cell carcinoma. As the disease progresses, it can cause a variety of symptoms related to metastasis to the brain, bones, liver, and/or lungs.

Evaluation

A thorough examination of the skin to identify any suspicious lesions or nodules, especially on sun-exposed areas such as the head, neck, and extremities is important in the diagnostic workup. A biopsy of the suspected lesion will provide histopathological distinctive features of Merkel cell carcinoma including characteristic neuroendocrine cells, the presence of cytokeratin 20, and neuroendocrine markers such as chromogranin A and synaptophysin. Merkel cell carcinoid usually spreads to the lymph nodes first. Therefore, in cases where the tumor has been confirmed, a sentinel lymph node biopsy may be performed. Imaging studies utilized to diagnose a Merkel cell tumor include CT and PET-CT scans that can assess the extent of the tumor and identify any potential extracutaneous disease.[27,29]

Treatment

Early surgical consultation is advised when Merkel cell is suspected by the clinicians. Surgical removal with wide local excision of the primary tumor is the standard of care treatment. Wide-field adjuvant radiation therapy is often used postoperatively to reduce the risk of recurrence. In cases of metastatic Merkel cell carcinoid, the use of chemotherapeutic regimens (anthracyclines, taxanes, etoposide, platinum-based) is indicated; however, it offers a median progression-free survival of months. These tumors often express programmed death-1 (PD-1) and programmed death-ligand 1 (PD-L1) targets that make immunotherapy an attractive option with data showing that up to half of advanced Merkel cell carcinoid cases respond to immunotherapy options such as anti-PD1 antibodies (pembrolizumab).[30–32]

DISCLOSURE

The authors have nothing to disclose.

REFERENCES

1. Klöppel G. Neuroendocrine Neoplasms: Dichotomy, Origin and Classifications. Visc Med 2017;33(5):324–30.
2. Raphael MJ, Chan DL, Law C, et al. Principles of diagnosis and management of neuroendocrine tumours. CMAJ (Can Med Assoc J) 2017;189(10):E398–404.
3. Yao JC, Hassan M, Phan A, et al. One hundred years after "carcinoid": epidemiology of and prognostic factors for neuroendocrine tumors in 35,825 cases in the United States. J Clin Oncol 2008;26(18):3063–72.

4. Ter-Minassian M, Chan JA, Hooshmand SM, et al. Clinical presentation, recurrence, and survival in patients with neuroendocrine tumors: results from a prospective institutional database. Endocr Relat Cancer 2013;20(2):187–96.
5. Harpole DH Jr, Feldman JM, Buchanan S, et al. Bronchial carcinoid tumors: a retrospective analysis of 126 patients. Ann Thorac Surg 1992;54(1):50–4 [discussion 54-5].
6. Fink G, Krelbaum T, Yellin A, et al. Pulmonary carcinoid: presentation, diagnosis, and outcome in 142 cases in Israel and review of 640 cases from the literature. Chest 2001;119(6):1647–51.
7. Saha S, Hoda S, Godfrey R, et al. Carcinoid tumors of the gastrointestinal tract: a 44-year experience. South Med J 1989;82(12):1501–5.
8. Onaitis MW, Kirshbom PM, Hayward TZ, et al. Gastrointestinal carcinoids: characterization by site of origin and hormone production. Ann Surg 2000;232(4):549–56.
9. Vinik AI, Silva MP, Woltering EA, et al. Biochemical testing for neuroendocrine tumors. Pancreas 2009;38(8):876–89.
10. Kahil ME, Brown H, Fred HL. The carcinoid crisis. Arch Intern Med 1964;114:26–8.
11. Singh S, Asa SL, Dey C, et al. Diagnosis and management of gastrointestinal neuroendocrine tumors: An evidence-based Canadian consensus. Cancer Treat Rev 2016;47:32–45.
12. Singh S, Dey C, Kennecke H, et al. Consensus Recommendations for the Diagnosis and Management of Pancreatic Neuroendocrine Tumors: Guidelines from a Canadian National Expert Group. Ann Surg Oncol 2015;22(8):2685–99.
13. Halfdanarson TR, Rabe KG, Rubin J, et al. Pancreatic neuroendocrine tumors (PNETs): incidence, prognosis and recent trend toward improved survival. Ann Oncol 2008;19(10):1727–33.
14. O'Grady HL, Conlon KC. Pancreatic neuroendocrine tumours. Eur J Surg Oncol 2008;34(3):324–32.
15. Pape UF, Berndt U, Müller-Nordhorn J, et al. Prognostic factors of long-term outcome in gastroenteropancreatic neuroendocrine tumours. Endocr Relat Cancer 2008;15(4):1083–97.
16. Falconi M, Eriksson B, Kaltsas G, et al. ENETS Consensus Guidelines Update for the Management of Patients with Functional Pancreatic Neuroendocrine Tumors and Non-Functional Pancreatic Neuroendocrine Tumors. Neuroendocrinology 2016;103(2):153–71.
17. Sherlock M, Scarsbrook A, Abbas A, et al. Adrenal Incidentaloma. Endocr Rev 2020;41(6):775–820.
18. Fassnacht M, Dekkers OM, Else T, et al. European Society of Endocrinology Clinical Practice Guidelines on the management of adrenocortical carcinoma in adults, in collaboration with the European Network for the Study of Adrenal Tumors. Eur J Endocrinol 2018;179(4):G1–46.
19. Libé R, Borget I, Ronchi CL, et al. Prognostic factors in stage III-IV adrenocortical carcinomas (ACC): an European Network for the Study of Adrenal Tumor (ENSAT) study. Ann Oncol 2015;26(10):2119–25.
20. Mayo-Smith WW, Song JH, Boland GL, et al. Management of Incidental Adrenal Masses: A White Paper of the ACR Incidental Findings Committee. J Am Coll Radiol 2017;14(8):1038–44.
21. Fassnacht M, Arlt W, Bancos I, et al. Management of adrenal incidentalomas: European Society of Endocrinology Clinical Practice Guideline in collaboration with

the European Network for the Study of Adrenal Tumors. Eur J Endocrinol 2016; 175(2):G1–34.

22. Antonio K, Valdez MMN, Mercado-Asis L, et al. Pheochromocytoma/paraganglioma: recent updates in genetics, biochemistry, immunohistochemistry, metabolomics, imaging and therapeutic options. Gland Surg 2020;9(1):105–23.

23. Guerrero MA, Schreinemakers JM, Vriens MR, et al. Clinical spectrum of pheochromocytoma. J Am Coll Surg 2009;209(6):727–32.

24. Plouin PF, Gimenez-Roqueplo AP. Initial work-up and long-term follow-up in patients with phaeochromocytomas and paragangliomas. Best Pract Res Clin Endocrinol Metabol 2006;20(3):421–34.

25. Lenders JW, Duh QY, Eisenhofer G, et al. Pheochromocytoma and paraganglioma: an endocrine society clinical practice guideline. J Clin Endocrinol Metab 2014;99(6):1915–42.

26. Cerqueira A, Seco T, Costa A, et al. Pheochromocytoma and Paraganglioma: A Review of Diagnosis, Management and Treatment of Rare Causes of Hypertension. Cureus 2020;12(5):e7969.

27. Kaae J, Hansen AV, Biggar RJ, et al. Merkel cell carcinoma: incidence, mortality, and risk of other cancers. J Natl Cancer Inst 2010;102(11):793–801.

28. Harms KL, Healy MA, Nghiem P, et al. Analysis of Prognostic Factors from 9387 Merkel Cell Carcinoma Cases Forms the Basis for the New 8th Edition AJCC Staging System. Ann Surg Oncol 2016;23(11):3564–71.

29. Becker JC, Stang A, DeCaprio JA, et al. Merkel cell carcinoma. Nat Rev Dis Prim 2017;3:17077.

30. Nghiem PT, Bhatia S, Lipson EJ, et al. PD-1 Blockade with Pembrolizumab in Advanced Merkel-Cell Carcinoma. N Engl J Med 2016;374(26):2542–52.

31. Paulson KG, Iyer JG, Blom A, et al. Systemic immune suppression predicts diminished Merkel cell carcinoma-specific survival independent of stage. J Invest Dermatol 2013;133(3):642–6.

32. Colunga A, Pulliam T, Nghiem P. Merkel cell carcinoma in the age of immunotherapy: facts and hopes. Clin Cancer Res 2018;24(9):2035–43.

Moving?

Make sure your subscription moves with you!

To notify us of your new address, find your **Clinics Account Number** (located on your mailing label above your name), and contact customer service at:

Email: journalscustomerservice-usa@elsevier.com

800-654-2452 (subscribers in the U.S. & Canada)
314-447-8871 (subscribers outside of the U.S. & Canada)

Fax number: 314-447-8029

Elsevier Health Sciences Division
Subscription Customer Service
3251 Riverport Lane
Maryland Heights, MO 63043

Printed and bound by CPI Group (UK) Ltd, Croydon, CR0 4YY

08/05/2025

01864751-0011